# MARATHON MOM

# MARATHON MOM

## *The Wife and Mother Running Book*

Linda Schreiber and JoAnne Stang

*Foreword by James F. Fixx*

HOUGHTON MIFFLIN COMPANY BOSTON 1980

*Library of Congress Cataloging in Publication Data*

Schreiber, Linda.
Marathon mom.
Bibliography: p.
1. Running. 2. Sports for women.
I. Stang, JoAnne, joint author. II. Title.
GV1061.S37 796.4'26 79-27123
ISBN 0-395-29135-6
ISBN 0-395-29136-4 pbk.

Printed in the United States of America

S 10 9 8 7 6 5 4 3 2 1

A portion of this book has appeared in *McCall's*.

*This book is for Jim & Arnold*
*— Samantha, Zachary, Amanda, Danielle, & Elisabeth —*
*and David & Deborah*

# Acknowledgments

We are very grateful for the invaluable help and interview time given by Gary A. Gallo, M.D.; Michael Giannone, D.P.M.; David Propp, M.A.; Michael H. Sacks, M.D.; and Mona M. Shangold, M.D.; and we thank all the women interviewed for this book — particularly Katie Baxter, Freya Block, Phyllis Cantor, Roslyn Capp, Denise Conlon, Mary Dono, Lois King, Mary Vitiello, and Donna Welsh. We're also indebted to Jeffrey B. Scanlan, Head of Information and Readers' Services at the Greenwich (Connecticut) Public Library, and the library staff; to Brigitte Bohy, Colette Conche, Lee Deubert, Michael Gallo, Douglas Heim, and Michael Quinn of the Fitness and Sports Conditioning Center of Greenwich, Connecticut; and to yoga instructor Sandy Heath and Mrs. Yvonne Covino.

This book would not have been possible without the help and encouragement of our husbands, Jim Schreiber and Arnold Stang, who did yeoman duty while we were writing.

# Foreword

One particularly malevolent winter dawn I was driving along a snowdrifted road in Greenwich, Connecticut, where Linda Schreiber and I both live. I was on my way to the airport and was none too pleased to be abroad on such a morning. As I negotiated a precarious twist in the road, trying not to slide to my final icy reward, the headlights picked out a female figure in black tights and running clothes. Oblivious to the weather, she was bobbing purposefully along at the edge of the pavement. On a day so forbidding that even the chickadees, those ornithological Eskimos, were no doubt huddling helpless and bewildered in their nests, this imperturbable woman was out running. As I got closer I saw that it was Linda.

Her appearance on that blustery morning seemed neatly symbolic of what has become of running. When I took my first steps a dozen or so years ago, just about the only people running were dedicated, long-time athletes. Toward the end of the 1970s, however, an increasing penetration of society began. First came businessmen, slipping off at lunchtime to YMCAs and parks to put in their miles. Then came vast masses of young men and women, convivially clogging Central Park, Golden Gate Park, and the running track at

UCLA, and in the process driving the nation's singles bars to the brink of bankruptcy. Surveys showed that perhaps 40,000,000 Americans had become regular runners.

The boom had not, however, caught everyone. Among the sedentary there remained a few men and women who for the very best of reasons could not set aside the time or did not have the freedom to run. Linda Schreiber, housewife and mother of five young children, had every right to be at the very top of this list. The care of children can be a tyranny, one that is no less relentless just because it is a loving one.

Yet for several years now Linda had been a daily runner. This book explains why. As she writes, "When I began running, I ran for solitude — to have a few moments alone. To my surprise I found a companion out on the road, a friend I'd lost track of during those busy years with the babies. That companion was *me*. I finally had time to slow down and listen to my own breathing, to hear my heart beat and my mind speak."

That's as persuasive a reason for running as I know of. One day, as I was reading the manuscript of *Marathon Mom,* I considered not running, or at the very least cutting my customary run short. The night before I had been out late, and I was paying a well-deserved price. Then, remembering Linda's example, I was embarrassed at my slothfulness. I put on my running shoes and went, thanking her. You will, too.

JAMES F. FIXX

# Contents

ONE

# BEGINNING

## *How a Nonathletic Mother of Five Became a Happy Runner*

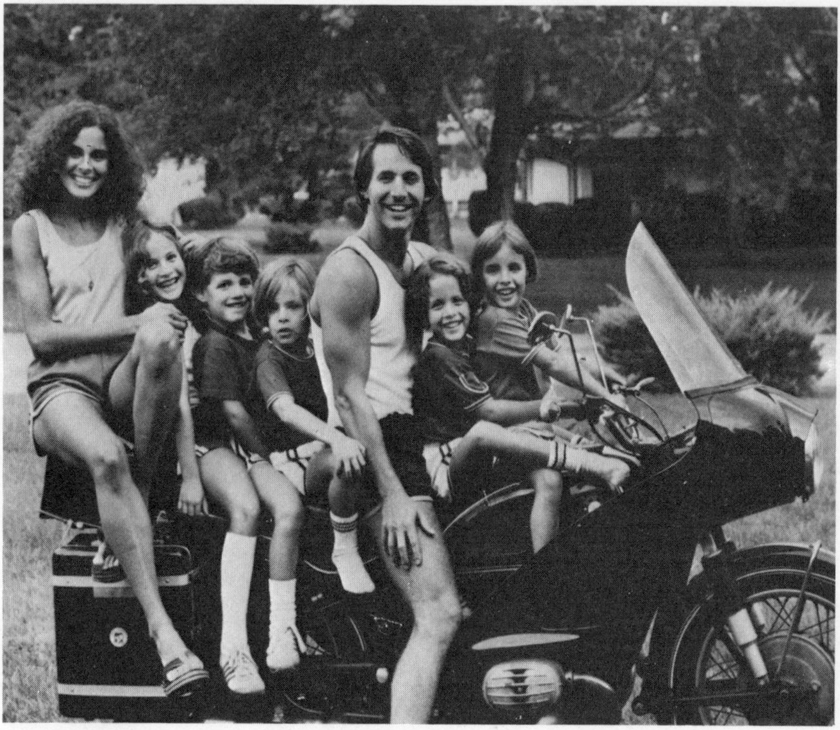

Tight squeeze behind the handlebars. (Left to right) Linda, Samantha, Zachary, Danielle, Jim, Amanda, and Elisabeth.
*Ken Regan, Camera 5*

I started running on a rainy Sunday in September 1974, and I remember the day vividly. My husband Jim was home — because of a canceled tennis game — and so were my children: Samantha, 4, and the quadruplets, Zachary, Danielle, Amanda, and Elisabeth. The quads were eighteen months old and in their usual fine form — singing, banging, pushing each other, and toddling into impossible places. They'd had no interest in napping that day, and I'd been watching them since 6 A.M. By early afternoon Jim and I had steered them through the major productions of baths, meals, and innumerable changes — wiping, hauling, consoling, and coddling. I'd also trotted through the domestic chores with unblinking and reflex precision: three beds made and four cribs stripped, five loads of laundry, a teetering pile of diapers folded, racks of bottles filled, food cooked, dishes stacked — plus mop-up and pick-up a thousand times over. Some nights the picking-up motions carried on into sleep, and I'd be snatching up toys in my dreams.

At some point I turned my back on the havoc to stare at the rain. Outwardly I tried to seem calm, but inwardly I was climbing the walls. I'd counted on good weather to give me a bit of a breather, even if that break was just sitting outside on the lawn with the children.

Jim must have sensed how I felt because he walked over to me and — out of the blue — suggested I go for a run. Athletics were an integral part of Jim's life, and two-mile runs and tennis games were usual weekend routines for him. The thought of a run surprised me at first, but then I thought "Why not?" So in painter's pants, sweatshirt, and tennis shoes I started off in the rain — not expecting much, but willing to see if a run would help me relax. I knew it would certainly offer some solitude.

As I ran I had time to reflect, wryly, on my limitations in this sport, or any other. I was the classic nonathlete — twenty-five years old before I even rode a bicycle. I swam in the summer, of course, and was exposed to the usual activities at summer camp. I'd also sporadically tried to play tennis. Jim had taught the game at country clubs when he was in law school and was patient teaching me, but I didn't have the time to spend hours plugging away at it. I'd learned to ride a bicycle in New York City after Samantha's birth, just to get *some* exercise, and biking was still something I did whenever I could.

*

The point in my life when I realized that my strength was sadly inadequate was just after the birth of the quads. We'd been told to expect four babies, so their number wasn't a surprise, but the arrival date was. At my doctor's insistence I'd gone to New York Hospital on December 1, 1972, even though the babies weren't due until February 20. The quads then astonished everyone by appearing seven weeks early, on December 30.

I knew right away that a month of enforced prenatal bed-rest was no preparation for such strenuous motherhood. Since the babies were premature, they were fed every three hours. I nursed them during the day and early evening, and they were tube-fed during the night. I spent the rest of my hospital stay rushing from my room in one building to the premature nursery on another floor in another wing. Getting home wasn't much of an improvement. We were lucky enough to have a nurse for the first three months, but the nurse's day off prompted weekly trauma. On those days I would hire a Barnard College student, just for that second pair of hands. One swore to me later that when she first stood on my threshold, I'd tossed her a baby, Fran Tarkenton-style.

We'd moved from New York City to Greenwich, Connecticut, in September 1973, and that first year in the suburbs had been rough. First, the babies came down with a sudden virus and had to be watched round-the-clock. The stress was incredible — and not just in terms of the feedings, changes, and the night duty that the illness generated. I was taking nurse's notes as well, so I could report accurately to the pediatrician. Keeping notes on one sick child is not so complicated, but if you're trying to report on a 24-hour period for four babies — all of whom are vomiting, have diarrhea, and seem to be on the verge of dehydration — it can be harrowing. I had a mother's helper at the time, and we were always going nonstop.

Then there was the day of the ice storm and power failure. We woke to find that the clocks had stopped and the house was freezing. Jim started a fire in the family room and we brought the babies downstairs. I had no help that day and Jim had to be in a New York court, arguing a case. He piled stacks of wood near the fireplace before he left, and the sound of the door closing behind him reminded me that I didn't know another soul in Greenwich to whom I could turn. I became an automaton — bundling the babies in extra sweaters, feeding them bottles and food warmed at the fireplace, piling on wood, and fighting panic. When Jim walked in at six I had the babies lined up in infant seats and was spoon-feeding them by candlelight. I gave him one of those overwrought smiles and thought I looked cheerful. He thought I looked desperate.

All of these worries were balanced, of course, by a

mother's normal pride and pleasure in the children's development. The quads by that time were a far cry from the mewling preemies in the hospital nursery. Their most distinctive characteristic, in fact, was the way they gained weight in leaps and bounds. I was aware of this when lifting them in and out of chairs, cars, and supermarket carts — a hundred pounds–plus of babies each time. I was thankful the children were flourishing — but mama was falling behind.

I was always tired and totally chained to the house. The big weekly events were trips to the nearby supermarket, drugstore, or pediatrician; and it was a year before I saw downtown Greenwich at all. I felt totally bogged down in routine and had no sense of my own existence.

*

So I ran that Sunday morning — because of a pervasive restlessness and because I wanted the solitude. I put one foot in front of the other, letting the rain dribble down my face, and I found that I was enjoying myself. When I got back to the house I felt breathless and muscle-tired — but exuberant. I was using my body in a different and demanding — yet satisfying — way. It was a totally novel experience, and I had a definite feeling of accomplishment. I ran the same two and a half miles a few more times that week, then I went to three miles. Within three weeks I was running virtually every day.

The things that made running attractive to me were simple and basic. First, it made me feel good — energized, exhilarated, and alive. Then I liked the efficiency and economy of it. Except for running shoes, it required no special equipment, and I only had to step out the door to begin. I found I could run right after we gave the quads breakfast and be back in twenty-five minutes. Running was an exercise system that kept me close to the house.

But the greatest initial benefit was simply the "time out."

In my busy establishment, there was no way I could have gone to another part of the house and done calisthenics or yoga for thirty minutes. The babies would have followed. In order to get a break, I had to get out.

Day after day as I ran, I began to realize that the running was beneficial in ways I'd never anticipated. Away from the hubbub at home, I was able to listen to what was going on inside my own mind. The thoughts and signals I'd blocked up — out of necessity — were all coming through again. I had time to reflect.

Each time I came back from a run, I felt I had done something good for myself, that I'd not allowed myself to be overwhelmed by all the functions I had to perform. I was exercising the right to be me, as well as the mother of five.

I loved my family and I knew all the chores were practical and essential, but I often felt overwhelmed by my life. I knew I needed space and time of my own — and running was giving me that. It provided me with a few private moments every day on a regular basis, and that private space enhanced my sense of personhood. Running released me and fulfilled me at the same time, so that I could resume the rest of my routine with equanimity.

I realized that if I hadn't gone running each morning, I would have drooped while doing the jobs at home. Now I whipped through them. There was a new feeling toward housework, an attitude of "Well, I got that done in pretty short order — that was pretty neat." It seemed appropriate to cool down from the run with some physical chores, rather than collapsing.

I was able to hop off the merry-go-round, then hop on again and go full speed around the circle. Now the boredom of laundry-dishwashing-bottles-bed-cleaning-and-meals didn't seem so frustrating, and I started the morning with a sense of accomplishment. I'd done more with that brief space of time than sit over the newspaper and a cup of coffee, postponing those jobs. I had more acceptance of the humdrum and there was real satisfaction in getting everything finished.

There was also dramatic improvement in my physical strength. The more I ran, the easier hauling groceries and carrying babies became. I found I had more pep, needed less sleep. Running also seemed to allow me to see things in a more mellow perspective, to make me more patient and tolerant. Jim noticed that I seemed better able to manage the kids single-handedly, and I had more energy for him when *he* came home. There'd been periods when he'd have a lot of exciting things to share, but I couldn't match his enthusiasm. I'd felt I hadn't much to contribute. Now I didn't feel so narrow and confined, because my day had at least included a run. Somehow I didn't feel so "small" and events at home so petty.

Running gave me confidence — a particular ease. No matter what happened during the day, I felt I could handle it. My runs went from three to five to seven miles a day over a two-year period, and I now generally run ten to twelve miles a day. I've run a succession of races and marathons too, including the 1977 Boston Marathon and the 1978 New York City Marathon, where I came in 11th in a field of 1100 women entrants with a time of 2:54:33.

Each mileage increase, each race completed, brought a tremendous sense of achievement. I had gotten in touch with my body again, and was testing its capabilities and its limits. The process increased my self-reliance and self-esteem unbelievably.

But the greatest boon has been the pure joy of the running experience — the feeling of peace and easing of tension as the run proceeds, the satisfying feel of the physical workout, the sense of pleasurable fatigue after pushing my body, the communion with wind, trees, and sky.

I love running. It has changed my life.

TWO

# WHY YOU HAVE THE RIGHT TO RUN

## *How to Find Your Own "Space" in the Day*

When I began to run I found I constantly felt guilty. The running itself made me feel wonderful — it rested my mind, strengthened my body, and only took twenty-five minutes a day. But I knew that whenever I wasn't home, extra burdens were put on whoever *was* there. Every morning when I spurted away from the house, I knew the mother's helper or sitter I left behind would be running double-time too, coping with the needs and demands of four active babies.

My feelings bothered me. Not during the run — the relief of the physical workout was such a pleasure that nothing could have diminished it. But the rest of the day, guilt gnawed at me. I knew it was silly. I was away at other times, too — marketing or driving Samantha to nursery school. But those were legitimate errands — running was something I *chose* to do.

Jim was supportive and tried to help me work out my feelings, but I couldn't shake off the idea that leaving someone else alone with the children was selfish. I'd come back from a run feeling energized and with a sense of wholeness again — then sort of crumple inside when I'd find my surrogate almost out of her depth. There's just so much to do for four infants.

Sometimes other people implied that my running was not only self-centered but strange. There weren't nearly so many runners in 1974, and most were men. When I'd try to describe particularly challenging runs to friends — runs in rain or snow, for instance — I'd get some distinctly odd looks. A chat over coffee would have been socially acceptable, but a 25-minute run seemed weird. I'm afraid the prevailing feeling was that something was out of joint — that the running activity was a crutch that enabled me to cope with my family responsibilities.

It did help me cope, of course, but not as a crutch. It helped by setting aside time in the day that belonged just to me. The *amount* of time was very small — too small for going back to school or holding a part-time job — but it was a way of place-holding, of affirming that one day I would be able to use the time in another way. I was holding out space to be me.

As soon as I recognized that fact in the only true way — emotionally — my guilt began to fade. But that was a year later and I was helped by the fact that the quads were then in nursery school. Still later, as I came to know other women runners, I wondered how much guilt *they'd* had to shoulder. The answer was . . . plenty. They knew they were engaging in a healthy and appropriate activity. They knew it took just a small portion of their day. But they'd felt — or were made to feel — self-centered and indulgent.

Gathering material for this book, I spoke to dozens of women who were fitting their running into busy lives — schedules that often had to blend heavy family responsibilities with jobs or graduate school. Running was important to them — they felt it gave them the strength and tranquility they needed to get through the day — but most admitted having to struggle initially with varying amounts of guilt. It annoyed them — it often puzzled them — but it was there.

*

The problem seems to relate to our culture's image of women, and women's image of themselves. Cultivating athletic skills and being in good physical shape is something most American boys take for granted. They grow up with sports. Until very recently, though, there was no assumption that American girls would share these activities. Unless they went to an all-girls school with an inspired athletic director, most girls got just token exposure to sports. The word "tomboy" is considered sexist now, but for years it was used to shame girls who competed as athletes on school playgrounds. They were considered unfeminine. Most of these girls were tenacious enough to persist through the lower grades — revved up by the sheer pleasure of playing and winning. Usually they succumbed to the prevalent cultural patterns in adolescence, when peer pressure and the "unfeminine" tag proved too much to handle in high school.

My own experience was typical. As a girl growing into young womanhood, I swam and joined in the usual summer camp sports, but I never enjoyed the vigor of fierce competition or the healthy "sweat" of a physical workout. Academics were stressed and athletics were considered irrelevant — they weren't something that could be used in writing papers or raising a family. No one actually kept me from sports, but there was no incentive to try them.

When athletics elude you in childhood, it's often hard to catch up. I went from college to marriage to graduate school to being a mother. That can keep you pretty busy, and it never occurred to me to use my spare time for anything but reading a book. Jim, on the other hand, was an athlete. Football, hockey, and tennis were his sports at school, and he plays tournament tennis now. He was just as busy as I was, but we both took for granted that he'd *find* the time for physical workouts.

This pattern was common in the marriages of the women runners I interviewed. Many had husbands who began running first, and they realized that the family had quickly adapted to preserving and respecting the husband's running time. The wives were filled with admiration for the men's discipline, but admitted some feelings of jealousy. Freya Block is an architectural designer and the mother of three who manages a career in Manhattan, a brownstone in Brooklyn, and a house in northwestern Connecticut. She runs six days a week.

"Before I started running myself I envied my husband," she said. "I saw that no matter how busy he was . . . how many problems he faced that day . . . he would *run.* I decided that if I managed to find the time and make the commitment, I would stick to it, too. I felt the running was a gift to myself."

Freya resolved her envy in a forthright way and got on with her running, but many women find this hard to do. Having spent their girlhoods in a culture that placed little value on athletics for women, they have no image of themselves as serious athletes and no confidence in their ability. Juggling the demands made on their time by modern wife-and-motherhood, and often competing in the professional or academic arena as well, they feel that private running time would be an impossible luxury — and a pointless one. Running and sports were activities for the rest of the family — the athletic ones.

The women I spoke to ran anyway — spurred by the desire for fitness, the example of a friend, or often sheer stubbornness. They ran — but guilt was their companion on the road. The fact is that a striking number of women do not feel they have the "right" to run.

The prevailing attitude is the traditional one: that *if* a woman has satisfactorily performed as wife-mother-homemaker-employee and finds any time left over, *then* she has the right to use that time as she chooses. But the "running time" rarely materialized. Mornings were hectic, the bulk of the day filled, evening crowded with cooking and children — and mother was pooped. To run out the door and down the street would have been an actual and symbolic departure. She'd be fleeing from pots in the sink while running toward a sense of herself as a person — and wouldn't that be the height of indulgence?

Just the contrary. I would never urge women to avoid their responsibilities, but sharing and compromise should also be part of family life. It's wrong for a woman to feel that she's only entitled to time for herself once her obligations are fulfilled — when they could be postponed for an hour, or some short cuts taken, or family members could help her with some of the jobs. I found this reluctance to speak up for "time out" cut through all backgrounds and incomes, from suburban housewives to $60,000-a-year executives. I talked to intelligent and perceptive women who found it hard to arrange the mechanics of their days so they would have twenty-five minutes for themselves.

I believe that women have a right to run for the same reason that men do — because they are human beings with a right to a certain space in the day that they can fill in their own way. This "space" is now more important than ever for both men and women, since our high-powered lifestyles subject both sexes to constant stress and stimulation.

Women runners who persisted found the running made a profound difference in their physical and emotional well-being — and had a healthy impact on their families as well. That's logical. If you have more strength, more zest, and do your work more efficiently, then you're bound to bring more spontaneity and patience to family relationships. As your fitness increases, your mind is tuned too.

Every life has its humdrum aspects, and it's easy to get bogged down in routine. Women are more subject to tedium since homemaking requires a repetition of tasks on a fairly strict time schedule. This can have a deadening effect on the creative energies. Women know the work they do is indispensable to their families, but when the chores are performed mechanically year after year they often find diminished satisfaction in them. Even the working woman comes home to find she must deal with marketing, cooking, cleaning, and laundry.

Running helps with day-to-day responsibilities. As your physical well-being increases, so do your running goals. As you meet these goals, your feelings of accomplishment and self-esteem grow. These good feelings prompt a certain tranquility and a greater tolerance for repetitious tasks — so your family benefits, in both direct and subtle ways.

Women who continue to run after getting through the beginning stages do so for a variety of reasons. For some it is the sheer physical pleasure, the "glow" of the workout, the triumph of pitting their bodies against particular goals and winning out. Others run to preserve a sense of themselves, to have a peaceful time for their thoughts to flow, to be free of the realities of their working day. Many use the time for problem-solving — for reflecting on family situations, making decisions, or simply planning their day.

And many run because it is wonderful to be able to play again. As the literature of running increases, there is evidence that the "diversionary" or play elements of the sport may provide its most healthful aspects. Dr. Michael Sacks, assistant professor of psychiatry at the New York Hospital–Cornell Medical College, believes that people who stick with running do so for the simple enjoyment of it. A marathon runner himself, Dr. Sacks says, "Most of us are wrapped up in hard work, in maintaining serious relationships and caring for our families. Running allows us to play. One can get a sense of adventure, of fantasy, of chance-taking in sport and play that is not allowed in real adult life."

So there are many reasons why women should run, but if you want to run with a mind as guilt-free as our culture permits, try to get the help of your family first. This minimizes the hassles and allows you to enjoy yourself from stride one.

When you make the announcement, you may get some startled looks. Even families that are involved in sports may not think of you as a runner. Their first question (silently expressed to themselves) will be: "Can she do it?" In more sedentary families the question (often expressed aloud) will be: "How much time will this take away from *us?*"

Both camps can be managed, but it takes some skill. First you must realize that both questions stem from a sense of alarm. Even though you are functioning perfectly well — and may even be playing tennis or skiing — running is perceived as a strenuous sport. Runners sweat, plod through marathons, fall exhausted. It's important to explain that you will be running only 20–25 minutes a day at first, right in the neighborhood, and that you don't expect to challenge the records. Explain that you plan to run at a fixed time every day, with minimum disruption to the family schedule. Say that if you find you like running, the time will increase. In that case your husband or children might occasionally have to feed themselves, feed the baby, feed the dog, or throw washing into the machine. That doesn't sound too extreme and the athletic or semiathletic family will usually say, "fine" — and then decide (silently) that you'll never stick to it.

The sedentary family may be harder to persuade. If your husband is a committed "armchair sport" he may feel threatened by the idea of your running, because he isn't very pleased with his own physical condition. Sedentary children don't see the point of it. Family feelings are apt to translate into statements like (husband): "Because you ran, dinner is late," or (children) "Because you ran, you couldn't take us to the library."

The mother of this kind of family is going to have a tougher time. She's going to have to stand her ground and assert her rights — not in a belligerent way, but in matter-of-fact tones. She should say, "I want to run. It just takes a short amount of time and it's very important to me. Some things may not get done on time, but they will get done eventually."

I believe that a woman who wants to run owes it to herself to try. Running may not present her with any world-shaking revelations about herself, but if she persists, it's bound to increase her self-esteem and physical well-being. For hundreds of thousands of women, running has been a powerful positive force — energizing them and giving them good feelings about themselves.

Making the commitment may be difficult. Psychiatrist-author-runner Dr. Thaddeus Kostrubala says the move into running requires "a leap of faith." That's true. Running will change your body, your lifestyle, your outlook, and will touch your innermost thoughts. That *has* to affect not only you, but your family.

I think your family will react as mine has — and be glad to have a stronger, happier, mellower wife and mother. Six months after I started to run I was going out one morning when the quads called after me, "Go-go Ma-ma." The babies I'd worried about leaving were cheering me on.

THREE

# THE TIME

## *How to Borrow and Steal It*

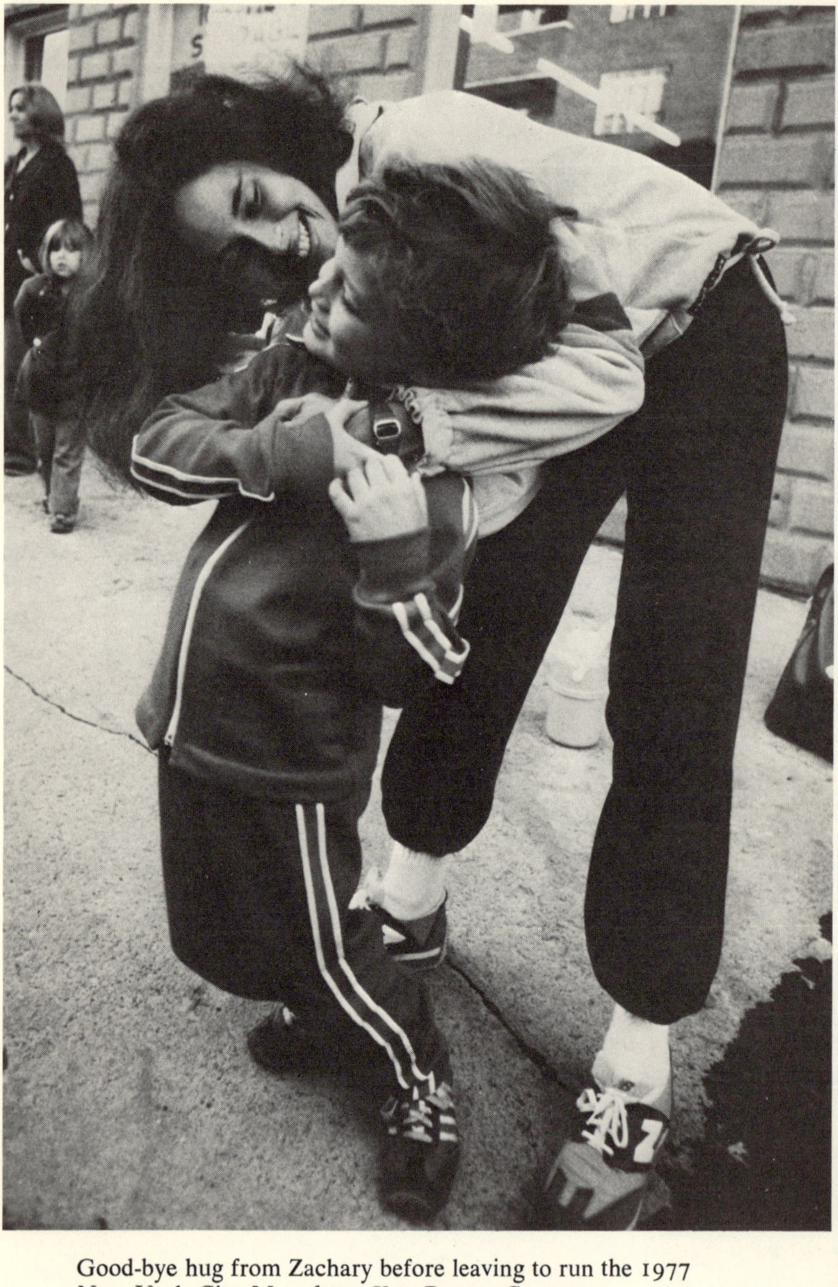

Good-bye hug from Zachary before leaving to run the 1977 New York City Marathon. *Ken Regan, Camera 5*

Time is the prime factor when you begin to run. Although your initial runs will be short, they should be firmly established in your day. Scheduling differs from woman to woman — there is no "right" time to run, as there's no "right" length of run, or "right" clothes to wear while running. Try to pick a time that fits best into your routine — a time when you feel energetic — and a time when running will do you the most good. This can sometimes be tricky, and the only way to find out what's best is to experiment.

When I began running my day started at 6 A.M. and ended at midnight. Jim and I would wake to the sound of the quads rocking their cribs to the center of the nursery, and fall into bed when preparations were finished for the following morning — diapers stacked, bottles filled, and laundry folded. Between those two poles, my free time was fragmentary — periodic segments of 10 or 20 minutes — barely long enough to catch my breath.

My first runs were snatched from that schedule, but when I'd progressed to three miles a day, they fell into a more regular pattern. I'd run every morning at 8:30 when the quads were finished with breakfast and content to play by themselves for a while. I ran right in the area, a mile or so in either direction, so my mother's helper could call me if I was needed. Six months later, when the babies played more self-reliantly, I increased my time to forty minutes and my distance to five miles.

I stayed at the five-mile point until the quads went to nursery school, and then the time period shifted again. I'd get up early, run seven miles from 7:15 to 8:15 and be back in time to dress the children and drive them to school by 9. They were only in school a few hours, and I found that if I didn't run early, I wouldn't run at all. I needed those school hours to market, do errands, and cope with debris.

When my mother's helper was gone on weekends, Jim would get up very early and run himself, then hold the fort while I ran. Sometimes we'd hire a sitter so we could run together, or we'd trade time — he'd sit while I ran, I'd sit while he played tennis. When we ran together we'd jog past our corner every fifteen minutes, so we could be flagged down if necessary.

Now the children are in elementary school full-time. We all get up about 7:15 and hustle through the breakfast and dressing routine. The school bus comes at 8:15 and the children just have to cross the street to get it. (They are their own queue.) I take care of a few domestic items, do some warm-up exercises, and then get out for my run.

I think women with young children will want to run early in the day — either before breakfast (while their husbands are still at home), or while the children are at school. If you let the run go until a later hour, the day tends to jam up and you may feel too fatigued. Besides, the average suburban mother spends her afternoons nailed to the driver's seat, shuttling children to their after-school activities.

Last year our Mondays were horrendous. Samantha met

with her Brownie troop at the civic center from 3 to 4:15, the younger girls had a dance class all the way across town from 4 to 5, Zachary swam at the Y from 4 to 4:45, and then Samantha had *her* dance class from 5 to 6. I would arrive home at 6:40 with five tired, cranky kids, and God help me if I didn't have dinner warming in the timed oven! My Monday morning runs were deposits in a patience-and-energy bank.

So through the years as the children grew and my running developed, I used different techniques to free the time. I had to fit running into the rigors of my own schedule — gauging the time available and accommodating the patterns of my running. Every woman has to do this for herself.

Almost all those I interviewed put together their running time by shaving minutes off something else. They slept a half-hour less or changed evening pastimes to get enough rest for the morning run — and noticed that the forfeited pastimes were usually sedentary ones. Some delegated jobs to cooperative husbands and families or simplified their housekeeping. The working women had already done some of this as a matter of course, but they had to pare down still further to fit runs into their busy days. Women who were caring for infants and children gathered time for their runs in ingenious ways.

Freya, whose job hours in Manhattan are 9 to 6, runs in a Brooklyn park for forty minutes, five days a week. The sixth day she runs on a path beside Connecticut's Housatonic River. Monday through Friday, she's up at 6:30, out by 6:40, and back in the house again by 7:20 after having run 2½ to 3½ miles, depending on her pace that day. Her husband, who also runs, gets up at 6:15, re-sets the alarm for her, and returns in time to start breakfast. (They pass in the park.) Between 7:20 and 8 A.M., Freya showers, dresses, makes the children's school lunches, and has her own breakfast. Her three children, 16, 13, and 10, leave for school at 8. After they're gone, Freya leaves herself, traveling forty minutes by subway to get to her office just before 9.

Freya is typical of many women who run but do not plan to increase their mileage and do not aspire to run races and marathons. Their running budget of thirty to forty minutes per day does the job for them. It keeps them fit physically and emotionally. As Freya says, "Running increases my energy level. If I don't run for any reason, I feel totally different during the day."

Phyllis Cantor is the director of library media services at the Greenwich High School and president of the Greenwich Education Association. The mother of four, her working day runs from 7:30 to 4 — but she must often return for long evening meetings. She runs from 6 to 6:30 A.M. and fits showering, dressing, and the twenty-minute drive to her office into the following hour. When she's out-of-town for business trips and conferences, she enjoys the morning run in new and different cities. One morning she had the pleasure of sprinting — in shorts — past an incredulous shift of Torrington, Connecticut, factory workers.

"Running puts me in charge of my day in several ways," Phyllis says. "It means little things . . . like getting out early to see what the weather is like, to know how to dress for the day. Running gives me time to ponder the problems I may have to confront, and the physical stamina I need for my work. If I run I feel bouncy all day . . . if I don't, I feel sluggish and stale."

Denise Conlon is a Greenwich mother of three who began running when her daughter was five months old. "I was heavy and feeling rather depleted after the baby's birth, and since I was nursing Danielle I was homebound as well. My husband ran and so did some of my friends. To slim down and for a change of pace, I decided to try it myself. There was no way I could leave the baby at that point, so I simply began running in circles outside the house." Now Denise runs three miles a day, five times a week. She's up and out by 5:30 A.M., and back just as the children are waking up. If there's a slight overlap and the baby wakes earlier, her husband is there to supervise. "I just feel refreshed and invigorated by running," Denise says, "and it helps me emotionally too. One afternoon when I was having a sticky time with the children, I walked out the door and ran in the rain. It was wonderful. I came back feeling relaxed . . . with my patience restored."

Katie Baxter's life is full — with husband, home, two children, and a Connecticut–New York commute to Fordham Law School. She has been running for six years. "My husband began just before I did, and he felt running did so much for him that he urged me to try. I really began for reasons of vanity . . . my second child was six months old, and I felt I was chunkier than I had to be. When I'm not training to race, I run an average of ten miles a week, but I find I have to vary the time. I don't run every morning at 8 A.M. . . . it's catch-as-catch-can.

"During the school year I'm committed to at least sixty hours' classroom work and study a week, which doesn't leave much time for anything else. So I sometimes run after I get off the train in the evening . . . mostly to let off steam . . . or I run in Central Park during a noon break at school. I change in the bathroom at Fordham and run out the front door in my shorts, past all the professors. At first people thought I was crazy, but now I'm just the girl who runs in the park."

Katie has run three marathons — the 1978 New York City Marathon, plus others in Vermont and Cleveland. She enjoys the excitement of races and the camaraderie that goes with them. "I love running where other people are running, which is why I enjoy Central Park so much. Running has made me much less inhibited about my body . . . I think nothing of dashing through the city in shorts. I'm physically healthier since I started to run, and much more relaxed."

Most of the women I spoke with had dealt imaginatively with time-and-place limitations before they evolved their own running systems. My friend Roslyn Capp began running when her three boys were little. She used the odometer on the family car to measure the driveway, and ran *there* for the first few months, while the children were napping. Another ran in place in her bedroom for eight weeks, so she could move on expertly to outdoor runs. One mother ran while her daughter biked beside her, and others have brought babies to tracks — with the stroller or baby corral placed clearly in view in track-center.

Some women have set up running groups and found they have both practical and social advantages. This works very simply. The group meets at a member's home, bringing their children. All of the members run except one, who sits with the children. The sitter-mother arranges *her* runs at home that week, with the help of her husband. The following week the sitter joins the running group, while another mother sits. The plan works particularly well with congenial neighborhood groups, who enjoy the sociability as much as the running.

Other mothers who wanted to run have found help through community organizations. Many YWCA and YWHA chapters throughout the country have running activities, and they often have unisex tracks. Running groups can be set up through PTA contacts, or through other civic and social organizations. Working women may find that their company already sponsors a running club. Concerned about the health of their employees, many large corporations now sponsor fitness programs with sports and exercise facilities right on the premises. These programs are usually directed by a trained exercise physiologist, and they almost always feature running as a prime fitness tool.

In general, the women found time to run by simplifying other parts of their lives. They cut out time-wasting frills and concentrated on what was essential. They persuaded their families to help and gave certain jobs to the children. One busy executive said that she had each of her four school-age children make dinner one night a week. She and her husband also cooked dinner once, and the seventh night the family went out to a restaurant — a treat for all. She reported that now she wasn't "bushed" every evening, got to bed earlier, could run at 6 A.M. with no trouble — and the children were turning into fine cooks!

In order to run you must set your own priorities. Some of the runners ran fifty miles or more a week — and some ran ten. *All* said they were pleased and excited by the physical and emotional benefits the running provided. So running doesn't have to take a large chunk of your day. Pick a time, pick a goal, and stick to both.

FOUR

# HOW TO GET STARTED

## *The First Runs— Gear, Weather, and Technique*

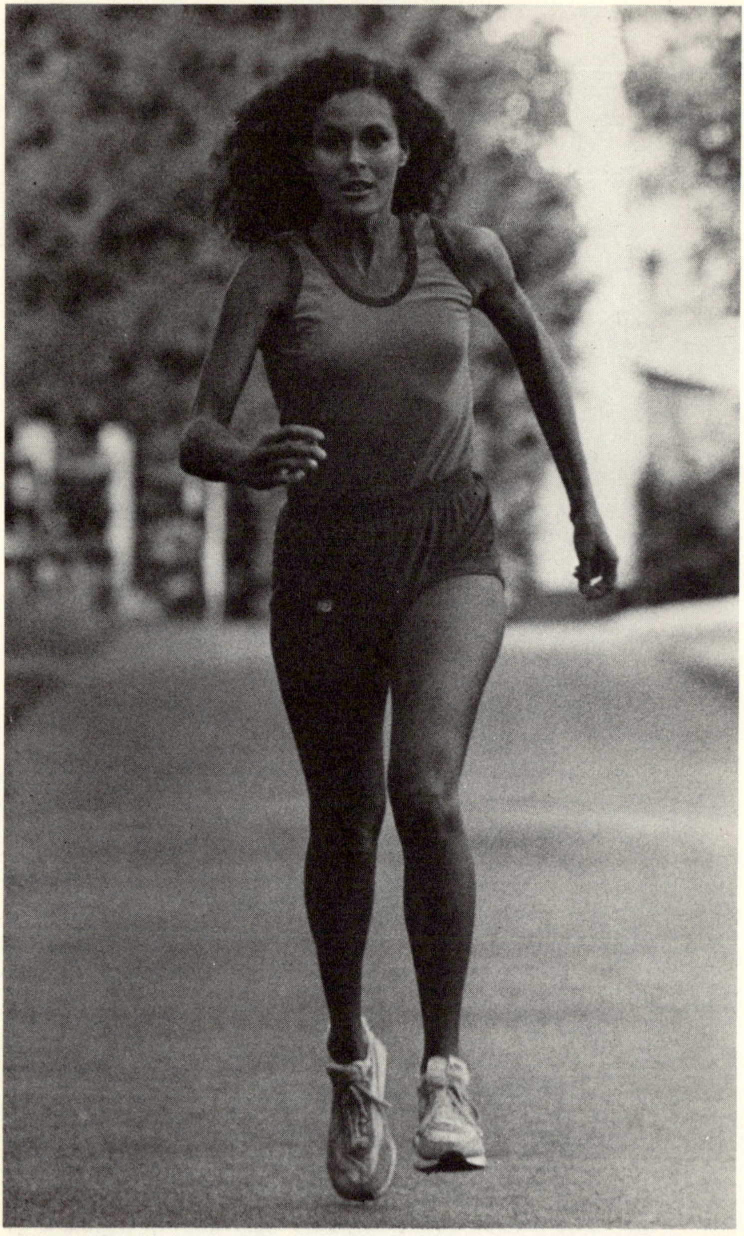

Getting into the rhythm of the run. *Melchior DiGiacomo*

When you've been running for a few months you may look back at the early period of floundering with amusement, and some puzzlement. It's so easy now — why did it seem so difficult then?

But some initial floundering is what everyone goes through. Unless you were born with winged feet or performed all your life as an athlete, a certain amount of shuffling and puffing can be expected those early weeks. As consolation, remind yourself that you're not alone.

The best way to succeed in running is to start out with some modest goals — goals compatible with your level of fitness and realistic in terms of the time you can spend on the effort. A good beginning plan might be to run twenty minutes a day — or every other day — then increase the time as your progress permits. Reaching these early goals will give you good feedback about yourself as a runner and encourage you to continue. Being unrealistic about what you can demand of your body is the quickest route to failure.

Make a commitment to yourself to try running for at least three months. The dirty word "discipline" enters here. It's discipline that will see you through the initial stages of running when a certain amount of aches, pains, and breathlessness can be expected. Once you make up your mind, keep to your plan. Try to run at the same time every day. Seasoned runners can juggle their sessions, but that's rarely successful in the beginning stages. Regular routine enforces the habit, so the daily run becomes a happy and permanent part of your day. I recommend stepping out in the morning and locking the door behind you. Once out, you will run — simply because backtracking seems foolish.

## Inhibitions

Don't be deterred by shyness. Although there are many more runners now, some women feel inhibited about getting out on the road. The degree of inhibition varies from those who feel shy the first time out, to women who actually get into cars and drive to secluded spots to run unobserved. They don't want anyone to see them looking clumsy, disheveled, or — God forbid — sweaty.

After I'd been running a short while, Jim and I took our annual one-week vacation in Bermuda. I was shy myself about running on the roads near the hotel, so I managed to do three miles daily on the hotel grounds, which was efficient, but dull. The following year I got out on the road and ran through Bermuda, gathering waves and smiles as I went, and really exploring. Now I do this whenever we go away from home — running is the best way to get the lay of the land wherever you may be.

Your running form may not be inspired at first, and you won't look your polished, best-groomed self while pounding along on the road, but who cares? As you are running, concentrate on the benefits being delivered to your health and psyche, and the inhibitions will gradually fade.

## Where to Run

After testing their full range of options, most people want to run outdoors. Indoor tracks have their points in really bad weather, for those who run on their lunch hour in city athletic clubs, and for mothers who must keep infants in sight when they exercise. Running in place indoors is helpful for those who simply cannot get out. Neither compares, in my estimation, with running outdoors.

Running under the trees and sky satisfies me in a basic, almost primitive, way. When the weather is good and I can contemplate my surroundings, I am putting myself in touch with nature. When the weather is bad, I'm pitting myself against the elements. Both experiences feed the spirit.

When you're running outdoors, your first consideration should be the surface underfoot. A common mistake of the novice runner is to think that the surface should be soft — lawn, verge, parkland, or golf course. Actually this is dangerous for the beginner, whose legs have not adapted to stress. Unless the grass you are running on is so superbly manicured that you can see every dimple and bump, you are much more likely to trip or turn an ankle in the natural pits of a grassy surface. I advise novices to stay off the grass until they've had some conditioning. I run on the black-top sidewalks and roads in my neighborhood. I like that surface, which is more resilient than city concrete, but I have friends who run on the streets with no problems at all.

If you want a safe, soft place to learn to run, a cinder track would probably be best, but they're not always easy to find. Most fair-sized cities maintain outdoor running trails or footpaths — usually in, or adjacent to, parkland. The most available track, however, will be the one at your local senior or junior high school. These are generally open to the public when they're not being used by the students. Parks and recreation departments give information on city tracks, and the local board of education can tell you about school tracks. A nearby college or university will probably also have a track you can use but, failing that, will surely have large expanses of on-campus sidewalks and roadways which can serve just as well.

There are divergent points of view about outdoor tracks. Most seasoned runners find them dull and infinitely prefer to "run free." Many beginners, however, feel very secure on them — mostly because of the sure surface underfoot and the absence of threats from cars, dogs, and hecklers. Which brings us to the subject of safety. I've never had an unhappy experience while running and, while luck may be a factor in this, I think what counts is my attitude. I run in a businesslike way. The road I use has a fair amount of traffic, so I stay on the sidewalk wherever I can. If I'm at a spot where there's no visibility because the road ahead is too hilly or curvy, I cross the street and run with traffic for that portion of the route. If you run on the same road at the same time every day, you'll get more friendly waves and nods than raucous hoots, since you'll have become a fixture in the lives of many motorists.

The rule to run by is: if in doubt, keep moving. Muggers rarely go for runners, because they know you can't be carrying much. If someone is following you with malicious intent, you'll have to outrun him anyway. The one exception to the rule is the four-footed friend — or enemy. Aggressive dogs are generally further excited if you continue to run, so it's better to stop and face them. If there's a handy stick or rock nearby, you might pick it up just in case, but if you see a dog patrolling his turf just ahead, it may be wise to cross the road. If confronted, my method is to face the dog and say in my deepest, most menacing tones, *"Go home!"* Most dogs are cowards and will obey you.

## Weather

I think it's a good idea to run in all kinds of weather, for several reasons. First, because it toughens you psychologically. Few things can compare with the inner core of self-sufficiency that comes with besting the elements. Running in bad weather also fuses you with *all* the faces of nature. Since every day can't unfold the shimmering lights of summer, it's a pleasure to see that bare trees in a snowy field and autumn leaves on a rain-slicked street have their own particular beauty.

Your most important reason, however, will be that you won't want to deprive yourself of the joy of a run because it is raining or snowing. I advise novices to go out in the first gentle rain they encounter as runners. If the weather is temperate, which it is most of the year in most of the United States, you'll find this is not an unpleasant experience. How wet you want to get on subsequent runs depends on personal inclination and mood. Some of my running friends would go out in snow but not in heavy rain — some loved the challenge of running in all weather conditions. I feel that thick whirling snowflakes and a soft cushion of snow underfoot can provide a delightful running experience, but I do draw the line at running in an ice storm, both when it's still raging and afterward. When the road is a sheet of ice it's simply too risky. On such days I try to get to the indoor track at the Y, or I skip rope in the garage.

Of all weather conditions, heat is the most dangerous for runners. Cold is a direct assault that you can cope with by wearing extra layers of clothing (see "What to Wear" below), but heat exhaustion is really treacherous because it sneaks up so rapidly. If it is above eighty degrees and fairly humid, be cautious. Try to run before 10 A.M. or after 4 P.M. If you can't do that, run in the shade and past water fountains, even if you have to change your route to do it. Drink plenty of water before you run, camel-fashion, and take more water or an electrolyte replacement beverage (Gatorade, or ERG) afterward. Use common sense. If you're out on a hot day and beginning to feel "played out" or crampy, stop running, rest, and then walk home.

## What to Wear

A friend of mine told me not long ago that — summer or winter — she only sees me in running shorts. (Not the same ones, I hasten to add, that I ran in that morning!) We laughed about that, and I admitted that running has had a pronounced effect on my wardrobe. I used to live in jeans or slacks, which seemed practical garb for the mother of five. Now I wear shorts — at least at home — and feel free and easy in them. I predict that at least *some* items of your running gear will creep into your regular wardrobe too. Running clothes are so comfortable that you'll resist getting out of them.

### *Shoes*

Sturdy, well-fitting running shoes are the runner's best ally. From the ankles up you can run in anything you like, weather permitting, but your feet must be properly shod. Can you run in sneakers or tennis shoes? The answer is emphatically *no.* Every time you take a running step, each foot must bear several times your body weight. The impact of each jolt is felt first by the muscles, ligaments, and the delicate bones of your feet — and is then carried up to your ankles, knees, and hips. This calls for shoes that fit properly and also support, balance, and cushion your feet.

A pair of running shoes can cost from $20 to over $40, but they're your *only* piece of equipment. With care and periodic repair, the shoes can last a year or two — especially if you later invest in a second pair and alternate them. Try to buy the shoes in a shop that has salespeople who are experienced in fitting running shoes. Generally department or discount-store personnel won't be as knowledgeable as those who work in a store that features sports and athletic equipment. It's best to buy shoes in the afternoon, because your feet usually swell in the course of the day. This is particularly true of women, who have a greater tendency to retain water. Have an understanding with the salesclerk that after the purchase you will want to wear the shoes briefly at home and if you feel they don't fit well after this test, you will return them.

Insist that the shoe clerk measure each foot individually, while you are standing up. The key measurements are:

(1) length from the heel to the longest toe,

(2) length from the heel to the ball of the foot at the widest point,

(3) width across the forefoot.

The most overlooked measurement is (2), which insures that the shoe will flex in the proper place. As for overall length, it's better to err on the side of too much rather than too little. A half-inch of extra room is not too much, considering that feet normally swell, particularly in summer heat. In winter any slack can be taken up by an extra pair of socks or an innersole, such as Dr. Scholl's lamb's wool-and-foam liner, which I routinely wear for extra warmth and cushioning. When you are having the shoes fitted, make sure you are wearing the socks you would normally use for running.

While you're in the store, test the shoes on these points:

(1) *The heel counter,* which is the solid piece of material built into the back of the heel, should be firm and amply padded. A heel counter that is too stiff and high can irritate the base of the Achilles tendon. The counter should grip your own heel snugly enough to stabilize it on landing and prevent excessive motion from being transmitted up the leg, where it may cause rotational injuries of the lower leg, knee, and hip. A heel counter that is too loose may cause blistering. Etonic brand shoes have a pre-shaped heel cup built into the shoe, which is a useful feature. Before the advent of women's models and width-sized training shoes, finding any with narrow heels was a real problem. Now there are many narrow-heeled women's models to choose from, but unfortunately many are also narrow in the front of the shoe, across the ball of the foot. This can squeeze the metatarsals and cause pain and cramping. My own experience with the women's models makes me feel they don't match their male counterparts in durability and shock absorption. For that reason I sometimes prefer the narrowest man's shoe I can find. I then "snug" the heel by cutting two sections of adhesive felt and applying one to either side of the heel inside the shoe. Sticking one piece of felt around the whole back doesn't do the same job and just shortens the shoe length.

(2) *The vamp,* which is the part of the shoe that covers the forefoot, should fit snugly. A vamp that is too loose can cause blisters. A too-tight vamp may squeeze the matatarsals and cause them to irritate the nerve endings between the toes — symptoms of this would be numbness, pain, and cramping of toes. The fit of the vamp is controlled by any one of three basic lacing systems: *U-throat* or *U-box* (full

lacing pattern down to toes), *vamp* or *Blucher* (laces across the instep only), and *speed lacing* (the laces pass through plastic or metal rings instead of eyelets on the shoe uppers). Speed lacing allows the laces to be pulled tight or loosened with a single tug anywhere along the laces — hence "speed" or "racing" laces. Dr. Michael Giannone, a Mount Kisco, New York, podiatrist who treats many runners, feels every running shoe should have at least 5 or 6 pairs of eyelets in order to be adjusted to an exact fit. He also advises against speed laces, because he feels they do not allow the tension to be adjusted as precisely as the conventional U-box arrangement. At least one prominent manufacturer appears to agree with him — the Brooks Company reverted to U-box from speed lacing in a recent "improved" model.

(3) *The toe box* is the vertical height from the insole to the shoe uppers in the shoe's front interior. The toe box should be roomy enough to permit you to wiggle your toes freely. Hold the shoe horizontally and check to see how the upper joins the sole at the toe end. It should rise up steeply, giving a snubbed and boxy appearance. A flat, sloping look generally means inadequate room for the toes. A lack of space in the toe box may cause calluses, corns, or damaged nails.

(4) *The sole* of the shoe is generally composed of three layers — outer sole, mid-sole, and insole. The outer sole is the bottom surface of the shoe, which hits the ground. It needs to be durable and must permit forefoot flexibility. Outer soles now come in an increasing variety of textures and patterns generally designed to promote good traction and to enhance wear. These vary from rippled and herringbone treads to waffle, hexagon, star, round-nub, and suction-cup types. The waffle types give excellent traction for cross-country running — but other than that, I have no special preference. The mid-sole is the additional layer of

cushioning material, which provides extra shock absorption. If the outer and mid-sole are too thick, they may create a platform effect that will cut the stability and efficiency of the shoe. The insole is the inner surface of the shoe, which comes in contact with the foot. Insoles may be made of leather, rubber, or a Spenco material, which has good shock-absorbing and friction-reducing properties. Spenco insoles come in all Nike shoes. Cloth insoles should be avoided. They are more irritating and they absorb and hold moisture. The total sole thickness should be higher under the heel than under the forefoot. This helps to avoid strain on the Achilles tendon.

(5) *The last* is the mold used by the manufacturer when producing the shoes. Unfortunately, some current shoes are modeled on a last that curves inward at the front of the shoe instead of being rounded. This is a poor design, since it unnecessarily constricts the forefoot and toe area.

(6) *The upper* is the nylon, leather, or suede top section of the shoe. Far more leather and suede running shoes used to be manufactured, but nylon seems the preferred material now. Leather and suede are warmer on cold, dry winter days but do not hold up well in bad weather. In rain, suede gets particularly heavy and waterlogged. Leather molds to the shape of the foot, thereby reinforcing and exaggerating any mechanical imperfections that may be present. I prefer either plain nylon or nylon or polyester mesh uppers. They wear extremely well, are light weight, retain their original shape, and are more flexible. Nylon absorbs water, as leather and suede do, but not nearly so much — and nylon dries faster. The nylon mesh has an additional advantage — it allows the foot to breathe and permits the evaporation of sweat, so you can run cooler in hot weather.

Several points about the care and repair of shoes: Maintenance is relatively simple — but should be done routinely to extend the life of the shoes. Nylon or polyester uppers may be cleaned with a mild detergent and water. Suede and leather should be allowed to air dry, brushed clean, and then shampooed with a special soap for suede and leather, which is available at shoe stores and shoe repair shops. Brush the soles of all types vigorously to clean out gravel, sand, and mud from between the ripples, nubs, or waffles. Extremely muddy shoes can be gently hosed (over a bucket or basin) in the kitchen sink with the sink hose, then allowed to dry.

A number of liquid rubber products are now available for the repair of tears and worn areas in all athletic shoes. In running shoes, the area of major wear is the sole — along the outer edge of the heel, across the ball of the foot, and to a lesser extent toward the toe end of the shoe. It's important to apply the rubber compound (Shoe Goo, Shoe Patch, etc.) before the area is excessively worn. Don't allow the outer sole to be worn through — once you wear down to the mid-sole, the shoe is hardly worth salvaging, since the mid-sole material is less durable than the outer sole.

Before you apply the repair liquid to the worn heel area, be sure the surface is clean and dry. Use the wood spatula provided (or a clean stick similar to a Popsicle stick) to level the material so it will be flush with the rest of the sole. Overbuilding the sole can be dangerous, since the elevated edge of the shoe is a smaller surface on which to land. The result is that the landing impact is not extended over the whole heel area, but concentrated along the repaired edge — and because the rubber product is harder than the sole material, less shock is absorbed. The increased shock is transmitted instead through the heel to the leg above, and can cause a stress fracture. The elevated edge can also pitch the foot so that it turns unnaturally, increasing the chance of strained ligaments and sprained ankles.

Dr. Giannone suggests an excellent method of insuring

that the repaired heel is perfectly level: apply the repair compound evenly over the worn area and then set the shoes right side up on a piece of waxed paper. When the shoes are dry, the waxed paper can be peeled off, and the surface will be smooth. Any excess around the edges can be trimmed away.

Sometimes you will buy a shoe that fits well but remains rather rigid. To increase flexibility, simply take a razor blade and slash three parallel lines across the outer sole at the widest part of the forefoot. The lines should be about one-quarter inch apart, and the depth of the outer sole. (The mid-sole material should be *just* visible through the slashes when you flex the shoe.) One has to summon up a certain amount of courage to do this with a new pair of shoes, but the trick really improves wear in the forefoot because it reduces the scraping and friction as your weight moves forward when you take off. Slashing the forefoot is especially helpful for women, since a 110-pound woman can't break in a new shoe as easily as a 160-pound man.

I think anyone planning to buy a pair of running shoes should check out the shoe ratings in *Runner's World*. The magazine annually (October issue) offers a detailed analysis of most of the popular training and racing flats. I also believe that every woman should give thought to the shoes she wears when she *isn't* running. High heels pitch you forward, shortening the calf muscles and putting a strain on the lower back. Runners should wear low heels on all but very special occasions. If you put feet that are used to running shoes into high heels, you may pull a muscle or tendon. Personally, high heels seem to me a throwback to bound feet in the way that they hobble women, and I have no use for a shoe that isn't comfortable. A final word on running shoes: if you find a pair that is really terrific, buy a second pair right away. If you wait too long, that model will probably be gone when you go back to the store — or the price will have risen.

*Socks*

Although some runners skip socks entirely, I don't advise this because I think it increases the chances of blistering. I prefer the orlon-blend, cushioned, pre-shaped sock (as opposed to tube socks) that are lined with stretch terry cloth. I sprinkle talcum powder in the front of my socks, then roll the talc back and distribute it in the heel area too. When I first started this practice I worried that perspiration would make the talc gummy, but this doesn't seem to happen. There's a little bit of beading, but there's also a silky-soft layer of talc that reduces the friction of the sock. Occasionally I also use anklet tennis socks, the kind with the roll collar or pompoms to keep the sock from pulling down.

*Bras*

Most physicians and gynecologists recommend wearing a bra while running, and many women seem to run more comfortably this way. Size is a factor — a large-breasted woman or a nursing mother certainly should wear a bra. I'm not so sure that bras are absolutely necessary for small-breasted women — but this, like many other aspects of running, falls into the realm of personal preference. If you do wear a bra, try to find one with wide straps and no metal — the kind with an elasticized back and no clasps. There are now new runners' bras on the market that fill the bill very well. Never run in a wired bra — the wiring can work itself out of the material and gash you; and never run in a bra that is constricting. While running you will want full inflation of the lungs, a diaphragm that is able to move, and a rib cage that can expand. A number of women, who prefer to be bra-less but want some support, wear a heavy stretch leotard or body stocking. I don't usually wear a bra for an everyday run — and I never do when racing. I find it limits my ability to breathe freely.

*General Gear*

I never wear fancy sweat suits with racing stripes and ankle zippers. It's also several years since I've worn sweat pants — they're warm in the winter, but they inevitably droop and get waterlogged in the rain. My standard outfit is a pair of shorts and a cotton or cotton-polyester T-shirt or turtleneck — and I add to or subtract from this according to the weather. I find the best shorts are side-split, nonbinding nylon or nylon knit types, preferably with a small pocket, which I find handy. Some shorts have inner lining pants, and at least one brand has mesh knit lining pants that allow for good circulation of air and are just about the coolest things you can wear on a hot day. In summer I replace the standard T-shirt with a tank top. I also wear a tennis-type wristlet for several reasons: I keep my key underneath it (looped on an elastic band); in summer it's nice for wiping off sweat; and in winter it keeps my wrists covered between sleeve-end and glove. When it rains I add a nylon shell and occasionally (in winter rain) I've resorted to a plain strapless bathing cap that I can tuck my hair into. I pull a knit hat over that. Obviously you will have to consider your hairdo a lost cause, but the object is to stay as warm and dry as possible.

In cold weather the first addition to the outfit is a pair of footless Danskin tights. I put my shorts and socks over these, and find them incredibly warm because of the close-to-the-body insulation. On sub-zero days I have worn two pairs of these tights and put knee socks over them. The tights are really fine for running — besides providing warmth, they're lightweight and shed water easily.

Layering of clothing is what keeps you warm in bitter weather, so when the temperature drops I wear a leotard, then a cotton T-shirt under a turtleneck, and a sweat shirt over that. It's good to have something warm around your neck so that the carotid artery isn't exposed to the cold. A turtleneck is ideal for this. If there's a stiff wind, I might put a nylon jacket or a down vest over all.

Since it's possible to get overheated while running even in the coldest weather, don't overdo, but be sure the vital points are covered. Wear a headband or knit cap over your ears. A knit cap is a good idea in any case; a large proportion of body heat is lost through the head. Gloves are essential to protect your hands. I tried down mittens first, but my hands were drenched with sweat when I wore them. I know mittens allow better conservation of body heat, but they also limit dexterity. I finally found that light woolen or ordinary cotton gloves work best, and I rub a nice creamy lotion into any chafed spots on my hands before putting them on. When the weather is brutally cold, you might consider adding two more items: a nylon mesh undershirt and a ski-mask. The undershirt became popular in Norway with cross-country skiers. It goes next to your skin, the mesh wicks away the perspiration, and you don't get chilled from a damp shirt. The one drawback to a leotard in cold weather is that it tends to trap perspiration in the small of the back. I always strip off my leotard as soon as I get home, to avoid chilling. When the temperature is hovering around zero, a ski-mask will protect your face from frostbite. Since wind is a big frostbite factor, the mask should also be worn even at somewhat warmer temperatures if a raw wind is blowing. The most familiar ski-masks are the gaily decorated wool or orlon types, but a silk knit mask can also be found in some ski shops. The silk masks have definite advantages — they're soft instead of scratchy and fold up like a handkerchief so they can be pulled out of a pocket if the weather worsens on your run. Although silk masks are harder to find, they're worth hunting for. When I bought mine, the saleswoman quipped, "There you are, dear. Don't wear it into the bank!"

In addition to basic gear you'll want stretch headbands to keep your hair back and some reflective tape or a reflective vest for running at night. The tape can be attached to the back of your shoes so headlights can pick it up. If I ran at night I would be sure to wear light-colored clothing topped with a reflective vest. There are now also Velcro-fastened bands for wrists, ankles, head, etc., made of reflective material.

The medical components of my gear include A & D ointment or petroleum jelly, Band-Aids, and Dr. Scholl's adhesive mole-foam, lamb's wool, and skin toughener. I discuss most of these further on, but I'll say here that petroleum jelly is the product most commonly used by runners to protect their skin. I use it on my lips daily to keep them from drying out, and on cold days I spread a thin film of it over my entire face. Petroleum jelly can be applied on the inside of the thighs, under the arms, in the crotch, on the nipples — or anywhere else where the friction of skin-on-skin or skin-on-clothing produces chafing.

## The First Runs

If you're not sure how fit you are, your first runs will tell you. Technically, fitness is the measurement of your body's strength, endurance, and flexibility. Do you participate in some sports — do a lot of walking or biking — or do you lead a generally sedentary life? Your initial runs should be tuned to your activity level.

I think your first goal should be simply to keep your body in motion for fifteen to twenty minutes. To do this you need not run the whole time — you can alternate running and walking, or simply walk the route very briskly. Do what feels comfortable. If this means you are doing more walking than running at first, that's fine. When you can run/walk for twenty minutes without too much exertion, your body will automatically shift gears and you'll just run.

When you begin, try to be relaxed. Think of your legs as light and springy and move your arms in counter-rhythm to the movement in your legs. Don't concern yourself with any particular running style, but do avoid a long-stretching or high-bounding stride. Arms, from shoulders to fingertips, should feel loose and relaxed, but your wrists and hands shouldn't be flopping. As you run, concentrate on keeping your body erect, and breathe naturally. That's all there is to it.

### *Huffing and Puffing*

I have to mention here that it's perfectly normal to be uncomfortable those first weeks on the road. You'll come back from the first runs feeling dragged out because your body has been strenuously exercised — perhaps for the first time in years. Stick with it, though. As you run more and more, the pains in your legs, the shortness of breath, and the fatigue will fade as your body learns to handle the distance it's going. This "breakthrough" varies from person to person, but gradually your run will seem to take less and less effort.

### *Speed*

When you are feeling entirely comfortable with twenty minutes on the road you may decide to build up your run. At that point increase the time — distance and speed will take care of themselves. Don't get hooked on a pattern of trying to go a little bit farther and a little bit faster each day. In the early stages, if you feel good and want to do more, just run for a longer time.

Many people who are perfectionists and "achievers" in other areas begin to apply rigid standards to their running. They feel the run is "wasted" if they haven't pushed themselves harder — or further — or faster. This is a sad way to run. It can reduce the joys and the benefits of the sport to a merely mechanical effort.

Your running should be unhassled, unhurried. You will want to wear an ordinary watch as a guide for increasing your time — for taking your pulse (see "Heart Rate" below) — or for practical reasons like getting back to an office or picking up children at school. Don't allow the watch to become a tyrant, however. Pushing your body to run too fast is a self-defeating activity.

The classic gauge of exertion level is the "talk test." If you are not too breathless to converse with a fellow runner, you're probably moving at the right pace. If you're running alone, reciting a poem or singing aloud will produce the same effect. Remember, the best barometer of how you're doing is how you feel. If your breathing is easier, your legs feel a lot lighter, and you are tuned into the rhythm of running — then you're making good progress.

### *Your Heart Rate*

Keeping tabs on your heart rate is another way of determining whether the pace you are running at is the best one for you. Actually three kinds of heart rates concern runners: maximum rate, resting rate, and training rate.

The formula for establishing the training rate is fairly simple. The maximum heart rate is roughly 220 per minute minus your age, so if you are twenty-five your maximum heart rate is 195 and if you are forty-five it's 175. Your resting heart rate is established by taking your pulse after sitting quietly for a few minutes. Your training rate is the resting heart rate, plus approximately 75 per cent of the difference between your resting and maximum heart rates. I say "approximately" because this varies according to the condition of the runner. If you smoke or are overweight, if you haven't exercised in many years or have had a recent illness, you should compute on a 65 per cent basis.

The formula, therefore, is this: subtract your resting heart rate from your maximum heart rate. Multiply the result by .75. Add *that* result to your resting heart rate. This should give you a target rate at which to train. (The Pulse Rate Table, Figure 1, in the Appendix will serve as a guideline.)

Your pulse can be felt either inside your wrist (avoid using your thumb, which has a pulse of its own), or on either side of your throat, just below your jaw. Practice finding your pulse, so it will be easy to count when you're on the road. To take it, use a watch with a second hand. Stop running, find the pulse, count the beat for six seconds, then add a zero. This will yield your actual pulse rate. If this is faster than the target rate for your age, you should slow down.

### *Precautions*

The current quantum leap into running is probably a worldwide rebellion against the level of "progress" that has made most of us sedentary creatures. People are running to get in touch with their bodies and to declare independence from the automobile, the armchair, and many of the tensions of modern life. Unfortunately, these have already had a stultifying impact on us. You've probably lost much of the fitness and physical verve you took for granted in your teens.

For this reason it's prudent to proceed with any vigorous exercise program cautiously. The average woman will have no problem with judicious amounts of carefully increased running. To be sure you're in shape to run, however, see your doctor for a thorough checkup. If you are over 30, he'll probably want you to have an electrocardiogram (EKG) to find out how your heart is functioning. If you are over forty or have any outstanding medical problems such as overweight, high blood pressure, diabetes, or heart disease — or a family history of such problems — your doctor will very likely want you to have an exercise stress test as well. This is a test designed to push your heart to work its hardest while it is being monitored for any functional irregularities by a physician. These are usually given at a hospital, but there are medical-testing organizations throughout the country that offer them as well. Be sure to follow your own doctor's recommendation about where to have the testing done. It's vitally important that the testing be performed under properly supervised conditions. If you are employed, your company may have an affiliation with an approved medical-testing group, and women with health insurance may find that their plan covers this testing.

*Warming Up*

Don't spring out the door until you do some warm-ups. Warm-ups are gentle exercises and stretches which limber up the muscles you'll be recruiting for your running. They prepare the heart muscle as well. Almost any moderately steady activity that elevates the heart rate above resting levels will serve to ease the transition from the resting state to strenuous exercise. It's important that the heart-lung machinery — which is so crucial to the body's system of energy delivery — be allowed a warm-up period so it can adapt to the high-energy demands of running.

Too many enthusiastic runners think of running as the "perfect exercise" and misguidedly assume that the "perfect warm-up" is more of the same. Nothing could be further from the truth. Running may be one of the most efficient ways to exercise the cardiovascular system, but it's far from the method of choice when it comes to exercising the musculoskeletal system.

Running uses the leg muscles very selectively. Running straight ahead is achieved by a repetition of the same series of muscular actions. The result is that the muscles that are worked get overworked — while the remaining muscles get a free ride. In the case of the distance runner, it's the muscles of the lower back and along the back of the leg that do most of the work. The hamstring, gastrocnemius, and soleus are the muscle groups that are repeatedly contracted, and in that process, tightened and shortened. These chronically tensed and shortened muscles have to be relaxed and stretched to prevent injury.

By contrast, the front muscle groups are little used by most distance runners. The runner with sore shins or aching quadriceps may argue that he's using these muscles (he can certainly feel them!), but actually these groups are seldom fully utilized, unless your training includes a lot of hills and speed work. If specific strengthening exercises are not done, the muscular development along the front of the leg remains weak. As the runner continues to train, the difference between the tight muscles along the back of the leg and the weak ones in front can cause an imbalance which leaves the runner prone to injury. It's ironic that many runners who pride themselves on their physical condition may fail to meet the minimum standards of flexibility that the desk-bound, nonathletic types can pass with ease. This was recently demonstrated (unabashedly) by outstanding marathoner Bill Rodgers. In an attempt to do a simple floor touch, he got hung up somewhere between his shins and ankles. Rodgers can get away with this, but less talented runners had better work at improving their flexibility.

The road to flexibility is (happily) no longer paved with strenuous calisthenics. Exercise physiologists now prefer slow and careful stretching to the old-fashioned bobble-and-bounce, and they even suggest that the conventional approach may do more harm than good. Many standard exercises increase the likelihood of overstretching, and overstretching activates the "stretch reflex." The "stretch reflex" is not a stretch at all, but a reflex *contraction* that is called into play to protect the muscles from injury whenever too much stretch is too forcefully applied. It's important to proper stretching to move *slowly* into the stretch, listening to your body all the while so that you can stop and hold the stretch position short of the point where stretching becomes *overstretching*. To pinpoint the degree of stretch accurately, you should assume the stretch position gradually and hold it (generally for 20–30 seconds) until you can evaluate the feedback from the tension of the stretch. If the stretch is within reasonable limits, the feeling of tension should diminish with time, as the muscles tire and then begin to relax and elongate. If the stretch is too extreme, the tension of the stretch increases as time passes, and the overstretched muscles are locked in contraction. Obviously such a tug-of-war does nothing for muscle flexibility. The following exercises are geared to counteracting the specific tightness problems that long distance runners experience:

(1) *The Wall Pushup* (rural version: tree pushup; domestic version: kitchen-counter pushup). Stand a few feet away from the wall, with one leg in front of the other, and lean against the wall with your hands or entire forearm. Bend the knee of the front leg; keep the rear knee locked and the rear foot pointing straight ahead with the heel on

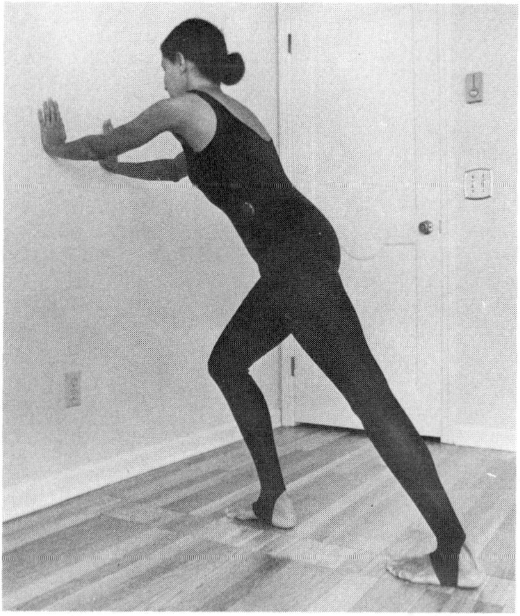

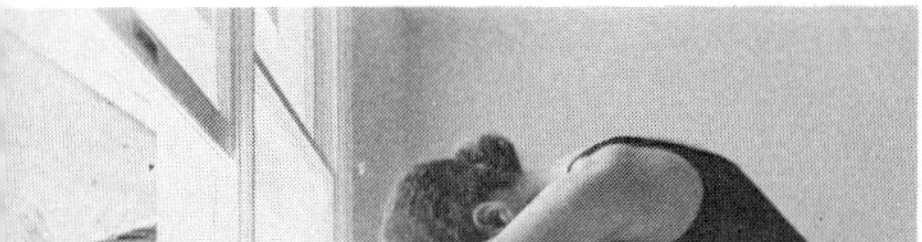

Wall pushup. See page 52.

Hamstring stretch variation.
See page 57.

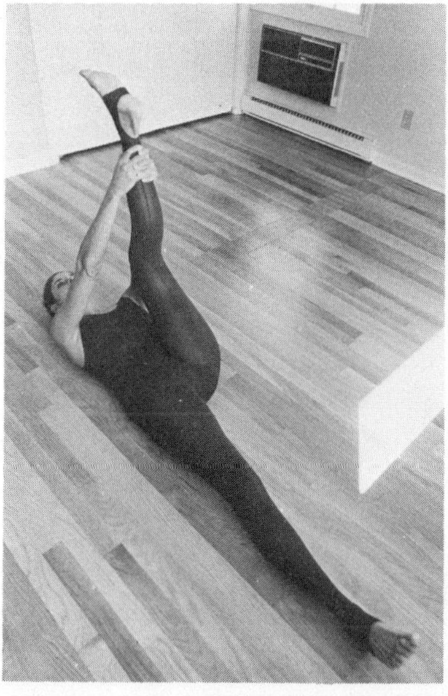

Hamstring stretch. See page 57.

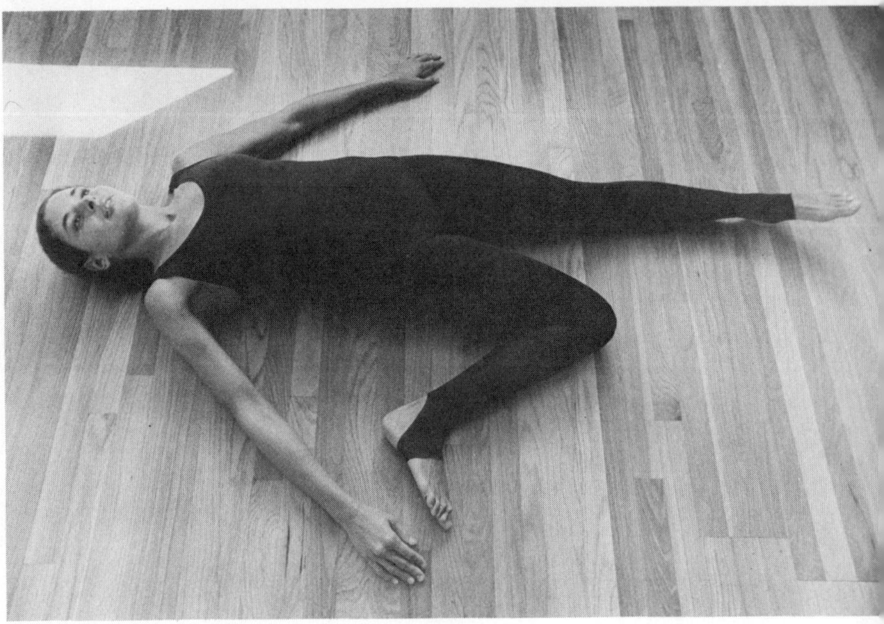

Quadriceps (or hurdler's) stretch. See page 57.

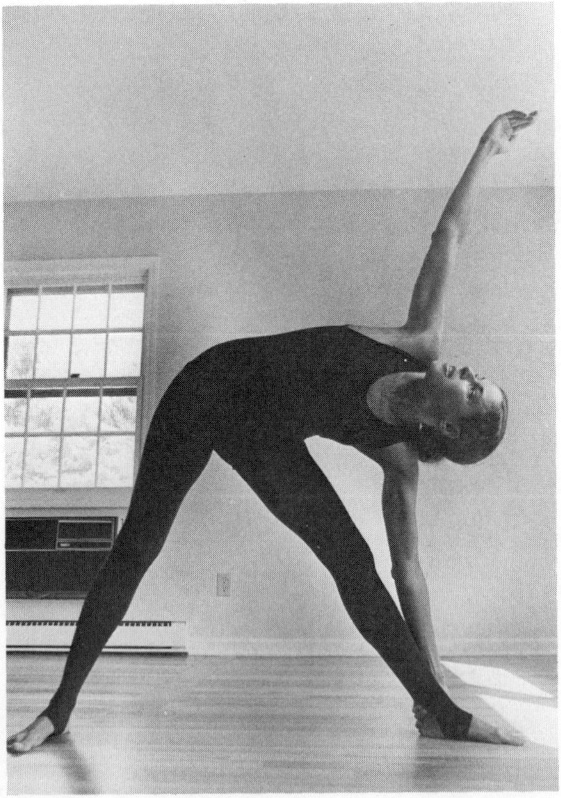

Triangle pose. See page 58.

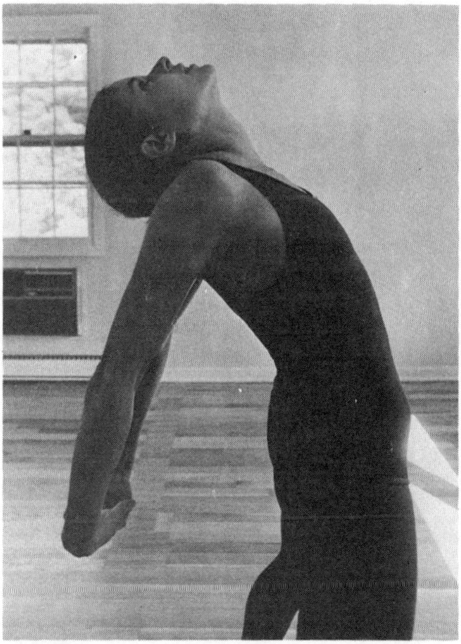

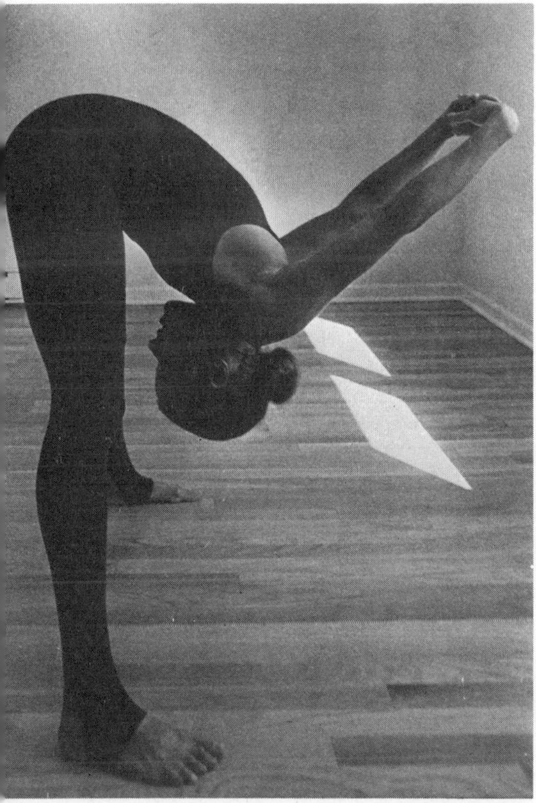

Chest expansion, position 1. See page 58.

Chest expansion, position 2. See page 58.

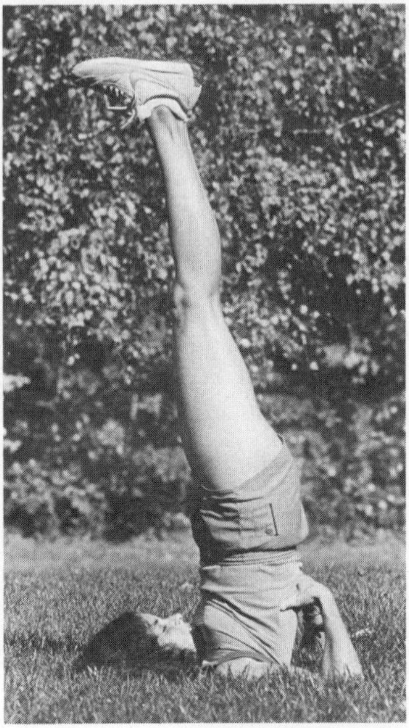

Shoulder stand. See page 58.

Plough. See page 58.

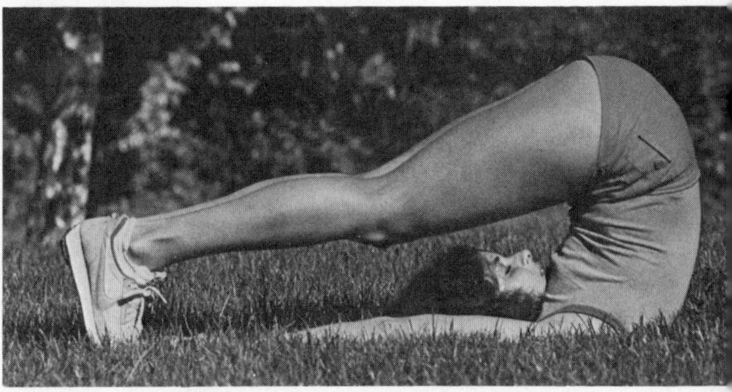

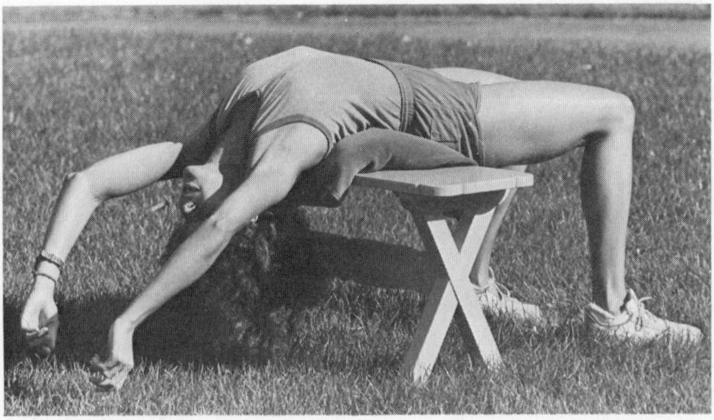

Rib-cage stretch
See page 80.

*All exercise ph*
*by Melchior*
*DiGiacomo*

the ground. Then move your hips toward the wall until the stretch is felt along the back of the knee and calf of the rear leg. Reverse legs and repeat.

*Variation:* By bending the knee of the rear leg, it's possible to concentrate the stretch in the region of the lower calf muscle and the Achilles tendon. Be sure the heel does not rise off the ground.

(2) *The Hamstring Stretch.* This classical ballet bar stretch for the hamstring can also be done with the back of a chair, a hurdle or fence, or even the hood of a car. Elevate the leg to be stretched on the bar; the support leg should be straight, with the foot pointed straight ahead. Lean forward from the waist, lowering your head toward your knee. Be sure to keep the knee of the raised leg straight. Hold 30 seconds or more. Repeat with the other leg.

*Variation:* The bar-less hamstring stretch. In the absence of suitable equipment, the hamstrings may be stretched by an alternate exercise. Lie flat on your back, legs extended straight. Raise one knee to your chest; the other leg remains flat. Grasp the raised leg with both hands just above the ankle and slowly raise and extend the leg until the knee is straight and the leg is vertical. Hold 30 seconds or more. As the tension abates, gently try to ease your raised leg forward toward your upper body. Hold again and release. Repeat with the other leg.

(3) *Quadriceps (or Hurdler's) Stretch.* Sit upright on the floor with one leg extended straight in front and the other leg bent behind you at the knee, with the heel as close to the hip as is comfortable. Gradually lower yourself down on your back as far as you can, supporting the upper body with your arms and making sure the small of the back is not arched off the ground. Hold 30 seconds or more; the body should feel relaxed.

*Variation:* This alternate is gentler on the knees. Lie on one side, resting your head on one arm. Bend your top leg back behind you and, with your free arm, grasp your foot, pulling it in toward your buttocks. Feel the stretch at the top of the thigh. Hold until the tension eases. Reverse sides and repeat.

(4) *The Triangle Pose.* Stand with your feet widely spaced, arms outstretched at your sides. Point the right foot out at a right angle. Bend to the right until your right hand reaches the floor (or gets as close as is comfortable). The left arm meanwhile points vertically straight, and your head is turned to follow the direction of your left arm. Stretch should be felt all along your left side (including the neck and waist) and (especially good for runners) along the inner thigh. Work up to holding this pose for 30 seconds or more. Switch the stance of your feet and bend to the opposite side.

(5) *The Chest Expansion.* This yoga exercise helps to open up the thoracic cavity and promote fuller inflation of the lungs. Clasp your hands together behind your back, interlace the fingers, and raise your arms high. First bend backward as far as possible, then forward as far as possible, head hanging, neck relaxed. Lift your arms as high as possible, bringing them forward over your lowered head. Bring your forehead to your knees.

(6) *The Shoulder Stand* and *The Plough.* Both are classical yoga poses and are extremely valuable to the runner. To do the shoulder stand, lie on your back with your legs stretched out. Roll your knees to your chest and with the same momentum, lift your hips and lower back off the floor, swinging your legs overhead. (In the classic yoga version, the legs are lifted straight from the hip.) Your elbows should be on the floor, as close together as possible, with your hands supporting your lower back. Straighten your

legs so that the legs and torso are in a straight vertical line and your big toes are directly above your eyes. To do the plough, drop your legs behind you until your toes touch the floor. Keep your elbows close together and your back as flat as possible, as if you were still in the shoulder stand. Both of these exercises should be done at first for 20–30 seconds, then the time gradually increased to five minutes or more as your flexibility improves. Many runners tend to roll directly over into the plough and never fully assume the shoulder stand, or don't stay in it long enough to experience its benefits. In addition to increasing the blood flow to the brain, the inverted position helps to reduce the sensation of pressure and puffiness that may develop after a hard training or racing effort when the legs are engorged with extra blood.

*Variations:* Instead of keeping your legs vertical, move them alternately backward and forward in a slow scissors-like motion. Gravity accentuates the stretch in the thighs. *Or* spread the legs as wide as possible (again gravity helps). Twist your body at the waist clockwise as far as possible and hold. Repeat, counterclockwise. Intense side stretch should be felt.

### *Cooling Down*

The point of a cool-down period is to help your heart and muscles gradually return to normal after a period of strenuous exertion. When you return from a run don't flop down to rest or jump into a hot shower. Walk around a bit or do some of your pre-run stretching exercises again. Your muscles are warmed up from the run, so they stretch easily, and the exercises will help undo any muscular tightening. Household jobs are also excellent "cool-downs" — making the beds or mopping the floor. Women running on their lunch hour can walk part-way back to the office. Just don't sit — keep moving for five or ten minutes.

*The Joy of the Run*

This chapter has concerned itself with the necessary details of running — tracks, shoes, tests, and exercises — but hasn't touched much on the joy of the sport. That pleasure you'll discover yourself. After the first difficult days have passed, there'll be one magic morning when you find you are sailing along in tune with your body — allied with the sun, sky, and earth. You'll feel playful and free and your mind will skim as fast as your feet. This is the essence of running, and it may be one of the most beautiful things life has to offer.

FIVE

# GETTING BETTER

## *Training, Running Clinics, Races, and Marathons*

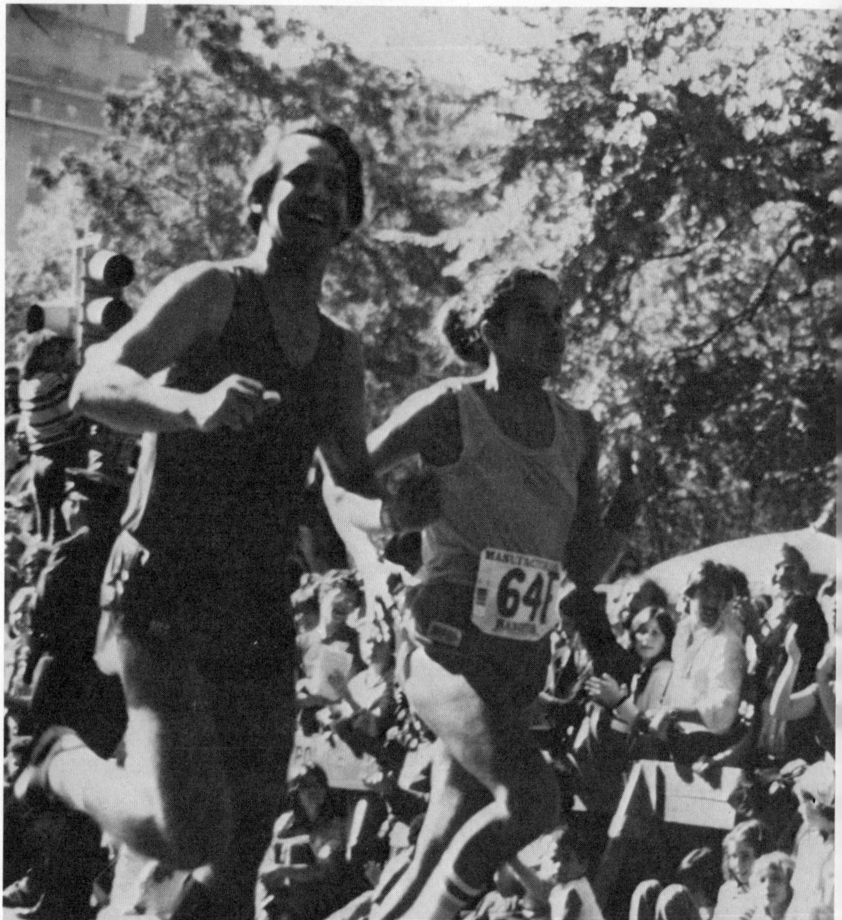

Approaching the finish line at the 1978 New York City Marathon. *Lloyd Hart*

My first race was a local Memorial Day five-miler in 1976, and I ran it like the classic novice — making every mistake in the book. The day began muggy and overcast — which should have been an omen — and I was hardly in tiptop shape. We were coping with a local siege of chicken pox (*very* local — six cases in just our family) and I'd had precious little sleep the night before. Jim, who was victim number four (numbers five and six broke out later that day), had planned to run himself, but his doctor forbade it. I thought I'd give it a try. After all, I'd been running for almost two years by myself; why not in a race with others?

Just before the start the haze disappeared, and the sun shone down full-blast. I started fairly well, but I knew I was in trouble before I was halfway through the course. My mouth seemed to be lined with cotton wool and my legs were leaden. The last half mile of the race was a long downhill run toward the finish on the high school track. I remember starting down the street gasping for air and feeling really winded and lightheaded. I remembered later that someone had physically stopped me — urging me to rest — and that I'd leaned on the hood of a car repeating, "I've got to keep running." I don't remember starting off again, or running the rest of the route. At the finish line I recall asking if anyone had seen a man with five children, then walking, nauseated and wobble-kneed, to the center of the track where I felt Jim would find me. And that's all I remember. I woke to find five anxious little faces hovering in a semicircle around me and someone holding water for me to sip. A friend came over, stared down at my prone body, and reported, "You just missed George Sheehan.* While you were out he took your pulse and said you'd be O.K." I finally got up and hobbled to the car with a worried Jim muttering, "That's strike one, Linda." He didn't have to say it. Just then I doubted if I'd *want* two more chances at racing. The day ended — typically — as a mixed bag. Stripping the children down for the kiddie pool we discovered the two other chicken-pox cases, and friends stopped by to deliver two trophies. The race hadn't been a complete fiasco after all — I'd come in first for local women, and eighth for women overall.

*

I sincerely hope that anyone facing her first race would not make as many foolish mistakes as I did. For the record, let me trot through them:

- In contemplating the race, I didn't take into account my lack of experience. As almost all my running had been done alone, I was unprepared for the amount of nervousness stirred by the thought of running with a group. I found that this apprehension was something I couldn't talk myself out of — and pre-race nervousness is a huge energy drain.
- Because the morning sky had been overcast — giving the

* The New Jersey cardiologist and runner who is the foremost philosopher of the sport.

illusion of coolness — I failed to appreciate how hot and humid the day really was. (More about hot weather training and racing further on.)

- I'd ignored all the rules for avoiding dehydration that I'd learned while raising the children (gleaned from a pediatrician who said the biggest problem in pediatrics was fluid management). Before the race, I'd been more concerned about lining up for the bathroom at the Y than taking a long drink of water.
- I was not in good physical condition because of my all-night stints with the chicken-pox victims.
- I ran compulsively. When that kindly spectator yanked me out of the field, I should have had the good sense to size up my condition and *stay* out.
- I set unrealistic goals in a race where I shouldn't have had any particular goals at all. Since I'd done the mileage before, I was overconfident and racing hard. A healthier approach to my first race would have been just to *run* it and ignore the competitive aspects.

So the mistakes were numcrous, but in my case somewhat understandable. Like most women who have been running for more than two or three years, I was a "self-starter." My mentor was my experience on the road, and my "experts" the few other runners I had met. I had no regular training companions — long-distance running was then a solitary and somewhat maverick endeavor. The only thing that wasn't haphazard about my training program was my consistency in sticking to it.

A woman beginning to run today has many more options available — from closely supervised Y-sponsored introductory running programs to the day-long or weekend workshops often sponsored by local colleges or running clubs. Another excellent guidance source is a running clinic. Running clinics are conducted throughout the country in various settings, and you can hunt them down through running organizations like the Road Runners Club of America or the National Jogging Association (see Running Clubs in the Appendix), your local Y, a nearby college, your high school athletic coach, or a local running club.

A well-conceived running clinic will present the techniques, psychology, and philosophy of running to participants on all levels of experience and ability. It will cover form and style, training techniques, injury prevention, and equipment selection, and will point out common errors, demonstrate various stretching exercises, and give flexibility tests so that runners can become aware of areas of tightness.

As a co-director of a running clinic held in the Fitness and Sports Conditioning Center of Greenwich during the summer of 1978, I worked with David Propp, whose ideas were important to my own development as a runner. David is a 1964 Olympic qualifier in the 400-meter hurdles and a world-class runner for the past 15 years who has competed in cross-country events in both the United States and Europe.

David believes that running should be free and expressive. He thinks that running goals should come from within, not in response to external pressures, and he says, "People shouldn't run the way they work . . . always achievement-oriented. I tell my students to find a way to run so the running is like dancing . . . or like singing a song. Enjoy your body in movement . . . immerse yourself in the flow and rhythm of the run. In running the means *is* the end."

Running for its own sake rather than for competition provides the training with more spontaneity. If the runner lets how she feels determine how far she'll run, and cherishes the element of playful abandonment, she'll get a lot out of the sport. She'll also stick with it. The running drop-out is usually someone who's pushing herself relentlessly.

The key, of course, is to remain in control of your running. That way you can race — or just run — as you choose, without feeling you have to prove yourself in either effort.

## Training Methods and Tips

All these warnings about rigid training regimens don't mean that the ideal running program is unstructured or haphazard. As in any other sport, running proficiency can be improved by purposeful training. It's helpful if you can train at least part of the time with a coach — as in a clinic situation — or if you can get out with an experienced runner who's willing to offer some guidance. The individual runner, however, can train herself very effectively with some basic knowledge of the common types of workouts.

*LSD — Long Slow Distance*

This is the most popular training method, and the one ideally suited to beginning runners. You are practicing long slow distance every time you run at a slow, even pace for the entire workout. LSD's greatest virtue is that it is an endurance activity of moderate intensity that is also the safest and most efficient way to improve your aerobic capacity. Your aerobic capacity refers to the maximum amount of oxygen that your body can process in a given time. The aerobic exercises — running, walking, bicycling, and swimming — are those that improve your ability to take in and deliver oxygen to your body tissues. If you can increase the amount of oxygen delivered and the efficiency of the delivery, then you can step up the body's burning of fuel with a resultant boost in energy. This translates into greater work capacity and better performance. It's the gain in aerobic capacity that is usually responsible for the beginner's improved sense of fitness. As your aerobic fitness increases, you can not only run farther but faster, because you are processing more oxygen.

*Interval Training*

Interval training is a method that features strenuous runs over a set distance with intervals of slow jogging or walking in between. If the aim of LSD is to allow you to run longer, the point of interval training is to get your body to tolerate a faster speed. The faster the pace — the shorter the in-between jogging distance — the more strenuous your interval workout will be. The distance and number of repetitions are determined by what distance the runner is trying to peak for in competition. A runner training for a marathon might do repeat miles, while a runner training for shorter events might do fast repeat 220s or 440s.*

Most interval training is done on a track, but a runner can also do short bursts of speed in the course of a long, continuous run — from street corner to corner or from one telephone pole to the next. This method allows the long distance runner to both improve her speed and vary her running routine. The drill approach to interval training — measured distance, timed speed, so many times around — focuses on nit-picking math instead of running pleasures.

Do some interval work if you're training for a race or want to reach some specific goal, but observe two precautions. First, warm up beforehand. Do at least 4–6 laps in a loose jog around the track and do careful stretching exercises as well. After the workout, jog slowly and stretch again, for a cool-down effect. Second, be sure your interval work doesn't exceed 5 per cent of your weekly mileage. If you go much higher than that, you're inviting chronic fatigue. Signs of overtraining (too much mileage, too much

*A "440" is 440 yards, or one circuit around a quarter-mile track. A "220" is, of course, half that distance.

speed, or both) are frequent colds, headaches, sore throats, swollen lymph nodes, tension, and a general lack of energy and enthusiasm for other activities. If your basal pulse rate (upon arising) is elevated ten beats or more per minute above your usual resting level, then you are either ill or overtraining.

*Fartlek*

This Swedish term means "speed-play" and explains itself. Fartlek incorporates the elements of a speed workout in an unstructured and flexible framework. Unlike interval training, which is usually done on a track, fartlek allows you to create your own map (literally) as you run different distances on different terrains. Starting off on a road, you might do short bursts of accelerations between mailboxes, then dart onto a trail in the woods or charge up a grassy slope, and jump over a stream before you head back. Fartlek gets you away from the humdrum, and keeps your running from going blah.

Fartlek's appeal is that it allows you to control the workout, while heightening your self-awareness. It also has another important practical advantage. "Because it encourages you to listen to your body before deciding how far and fast to run," David Propp says, "fartlek training can help avoid injury. If you're locked into a rigid routine calling for a hard set of intervals, you may overlook a genuine physical complaint in the interest of keeping to schedule. As a result, a minor tear incurred in the previous day of training might become a full-blown injury."

Fartlek also balances LSD's limitations. Psychologically, the fixed long distance schedule can become monotonous, but LSD has some physical drawbacks as well. If you run at an unvarying pace in an unvarying style on the same route, you're not getting an adequate overall adaptation of the musculoskeletal system. Many runners who have great strength and endurance when running in a straight line commonly injure themselves if they have to shift or pivot. The essence of fartlek training is variety in the workouts. Try to use different muscles and explore different ways of moving; periodically change your pace and route to vary the terrain. Your runs will become more expressive, and the variety will enhance your enjoyment.

Whether from sheer laziness or lack of ingenuity, my own running relies largely on LSD. I had no formal introduction to running or knowledge of training methods, and initially the thought of going to a track seemed foreign to me. A track represented a whole different world of athletics and competition. It was an arena in which I felt very unsure of myself.

So I built my training on a foundation of long slow distance. As I improved I simply increased the L in LSD and noticed (with surprise) that the S in LSD wasn't so slow after all. (I'm still amazed that the utter simplicity of putting one foot in front of the other can deliver such striking results.) At that point my running benefits were not purely physical. Running was a mellowing experience for me — a low-key, relaxed, and almost mindless pursuit. It was enough for me just to get out the door and be moving; variety and technique could wait.

Even now, I find it's hard to break the long slow distance habit, but I do try to vary my workouts by seeking different kinds of routes. You can do the same. Map out some hilly routes to run on days when you feel particularly energetic — push hard going up and coast down to recover. Or you can try David Propp's suggestion: *Don't* slow down as you go over the crest of a hill, but maintain the same pace for about 30 yards before slackening off. It's a revelation to discover that you can push yourself to go up and over the crest without stopping. This hill technique works physically and psychologically: it trains your body to handle the hills and recover more easily — and taking the hills nonstop is a great confidence booster.

You can also vary your LSD runs by changing the surface. Get off the paved surface and find a dirt path in a park, or run on a smooth, grassy verge. Try running around the edges of golf courses or on local beaches. Don't overlook area high schools and universities — many have cross-country courses as well as tracks. Check out local corporations — many suburban-based companies have built fitness trails for their employees, and some may also be used by area residents. Altering distance and pace will also bring variety to LSD runs, as will this straightforward but effective maneuver: to introduce speed elements into a basic LSD workout, simply run the last mile or half mile at a hard pace. (Follow this with a thorough cool-down at home.) This technique should insure that at least 5 per cent of your total mileage is speed work.

As you find some pattern emerging from your workouts, remember one basic training principle: the hard-easy rule. Alternate the intensity of your workouts, so that a hard run one day is followed by a lighter one the next. Your body needs those in-between days both to recover from stress and to grow stronger. Muscles, tendons, ligaments, and even bones can be weakened by cumulative stress and then become vulnerable to serious injury. Recovery days are a good time for doing your standard LSD workout.

Of course, all these variations will eventually stretch the LSD concept, but it's probably healthier to be less of a purist in that respect. The more your LSD training borders on fartlek, the more effectively LSD will serve as the basis of a well-rounded running program.

### *The Running Log*

You'll want to be able to measure your runs, to know how much distance you've covered each day. On a track this is easy — most are one quarter of a mile long, and you count the laps. Other courses can be measured by traveling over them by car, or on a bicycle, with an odometer. Keep a record of the mileage you cover in a running log — which can be something as simple as a small spiral notebook. Mark the date, how far you ran, where you ran, how long it took you (wear a watch but don't be a slave to it), what the weather was like, and anything else you'd like to include. When you flip through the book, month-by-month, you'll have a tangible record of your progress.

### *Form and Style*

Running is a natural motion, but the novice runner is seldom relaxed enough to move forward with ease. The rigidity is often not biomechanical, but psychological — and common signs are clenched fists, locked elbows, and (with women especially) arms that are carried too high. *Relax.* Keep your back straight unless you are sprinting, climbing a hill, or leaning into the wind. Avoid high-bounding strides and both constricted and exaggerated arm motions. Then think of yourself as a child running over an open field — and enjoy yourself.

## Races and Marathons

As your running gets better, you'll begin to think about racing. The decision to race is purely personal. Racing isn't a necessary extension of getting better, but if you're at the point where racing feels like a *natural expression* of your running progress, then go ahead and race.

Women race for the same reasons as men — they want to explore their limits, discover how far and how fast they can go, and rise to the competitive challenge. Competition forces you to challenge yourself in a way that running by yourself cannot.

The fact that women compete in distance events is taken for granted now, but just a few years ago the picture was totally different. The historic position of the female as the "weaker sex" led conservative medical and sports authorities to limit women's events to a half mile or less (though short sprints actually take more muscle power than long distance running). The modern woman runner is just a stride removed from the pioneer days of the women's running movement, which began when a woman ran the 1966 Boston Marathon for the first time. The woman was Roberta Gibb Bingay, who'd viewed the 1965 marathon with enthusiasm and decided to run the following year. When she was denied entrance (on the grounds that she might be injured), Roberta made her own arrangements. She hid in some bushes at the starting point, took off at the sound of the opening gun, and finished in a very respectable 3:21. Unofficially, of course — but she'd made her mark.

The following year Kathy Switzer signed her marathon entry form "K. V. Switzer" and took off for Boston with the rest of the pack. It was a cold, rainy day so Kathy's bulky sweat suit and hooded sweat shirt doubled effectively as a disguise. She was discovered four miles into the race and after some harrowing pull-and-tug with a marathon official, went on to finish in 4:20. She was then suspended from further competition by the Amateur Athletic Union on grounds of fraudulent entry (although dozens of men had also used their initials on the entry forms) and because she had run the race "without a chaperone." Since the struggle during the run was done in full view of the press truck, the incident got wide national coverage. It was the prime reason for heightened public awareness of the discriminatory AAU policy — and it reinforced the determination of the women runners. Many women now running their own first marathons have a sense of vicarious participation in that maiden voyage.

In the 1971 New York City Marathon, both Beth Bonner and Nina Kuscsik broke the 3-hour barrier and in doing so also broke the official AAU barrier — the following year the Boston Marathon was opened to women contestants. As women all over the country began having official numbers pinned on their T-shirts, the pressure to perform as symbols of their sex was replaced by eagerness to excel as individual competing athletes. The fact that women are becoming more competitive among themselves is clearly reflected in the way they are knocking down records at distance events — from the mile to the marathon.

Ironically, the reward of this progress has been an increase in the same "performance anxiety" that commonly afflicts men. This fear of failure points up a paradox in women's running today: women runners want to compete as freely and tenaciously as the men, but are often too inhibited to do so. The inhibitions exist partly because the athletic experience is a new one for many women, and partly because they have been culturally conditioned to regard most forms of competition as unfeminine.

The way this translates to running was illustrated by an acquaintance who was recently involved in her first race. As she was running the last mile she saw that if she could pass two women ahead of her, she would have a clear path to the finish line. She sprinted ahead and passed one of the women, but as she came abreast of the other, she turned and called out, "Come on!" Spurred by that encouragement, the second woman took off and finished first, leaving my friend chagrined. She realized the incident had happened because she was uncomfortable about being competitive. Women can overcome this ambivalence, and racing experience helps. So does the example set by record-breaking women runners — all of whom are successful (and unflappable) competitors.

If you want to explore the range of your running abilities, to see how far you can extend yourself — by all means race. Just remember that you can also enjoy participating in races on a low-key basis as a "fun runner." It's a great revelation to many runners that racing can be more shared experience than contest, and that there's a very strong sense of community in the midst of a racing group. Many women who race regularly do not do so competitively, but for the joy of this sharing.

Some of my friends, however, have absolutely no interest in racing. One frankly said, "I feel good about myself when I run. Some runs are better, some worse, but a run always sets me up and gives me extra energy. If I made the effort to race and didn't do well, that might destroy the good feeling I have about my running. I might not be as relaxed."

My advice is to follow your instincts and do exactly what you prefer. No one should feel defensive if she doesn't care to race. Having the freedom to race doesn't mean you're *obliged* to compete.

### *Getting Ready to Race*

For your first effort, pick a race that's manageable for you — one that relates to your training distance. This doesn't mean that if you plan to run a 10-km. race (6.2 miles) you must average that distance in your daily workout, but you should certainly run that far at least once. If you generally run in the 2–4-mile range, work a few 5- or 6-mile runs into your regular training before the race date. If this means building up your weekly mileage, try to do it at least a month in advance. A sudden, sharp increase in mileage (particularly at a faster pace) may cause an injury that can sideline you on the day of the race.

During this preparation period, it's a good idea to devote extra time to stretching exercises. You may find your muscles are especially tight at this time because you are running more miles and running them harder. You may also have a case of the pre-race jitters, which can translate into muscular tension. Concentrated daily stretching helps with both of these problems, and yoga stretches are particularly good because they promote deeper breathing and greater relaxation. The increased flexibility you'll gain will enhance your racing condition and provide extra protection against injury.

Though there's no way to duplicate all the conditions of the actual race beforehand, there *are* things you can do to familiarize yourself with what you may encounter. Wear a watch on your training runs to check your time. (A fancy stopwatch isn't necessary, but a second hand helps.) To calculate your average pace, clock the time of the run and divide by the distance. It's important to know whether you can sustain that training pace for the full race distance, so if you computed on a 3-mile basis, check yourself on a 6-mile run as well. (Chances are you'll be slower.) Try to maintain an even pace during these training runs. Tune into this pace and develop a feel for it — the arm swing, stride, tempo, and rhythm. You'll want to be able to find this pace and stay with it during the race.

If the race is a local one, check out the course beforehand. Cover it on foot first, running it once or twice in training. Then drive over the course to pinpoint several "landmarks" which you can use as distance markers. If you know these intermediate distances and your intended running pace, you can project how long it would take you to run from point to point. This is especially useful in a longer race where time splits are not announced, allowing you to judge whether you are running faster or slower than your target rate.

You should also consider sleeping and eating requirements — racing definitely affects your nutritional needs and patterns of rest. In running, "rest" is an overall term which means not just sleeping more, but training less. Your needs will really depend on the length of the event and the degree of racing effort. Certainly reasonable amounts of rest are important before any event — you shouldn't subject an already stressed body to the additional pressures of racing.

There's some controversy about the idea of making diet changes before a race. I don't feel a special pre-race diet is important unless your effort will approach marathon distance — 20 miles at least. For a marathon (or ultramarathon)* some runners prefer the carbohydrate-loading technique.

A carbohydrate-loading regimen should begin one week before the big race, and is preceded by a long, *slow* depletion run of 15 or 20 miles. The idea of the run is to burn any residual stores of carbohydrates that the body has in reserve. The diet that follows the run then uses up whatever carbohydrates remain (stored in the liver and the muscle tissues in the form of glycogen). On the first three days of the pre-race week, the runner sticks to a diet in which there are virtually no carbohydrates, such as grains, starches, fruits, sweets, and baked goods (vegetables are also kept to a minimum). Protein should be eaten instead — meat, chicken, fish, cheese, and eggs, plus some fats — all of these in *small amounts*. This is the carbohydrate-depletion

* A marathon is a race of 26.2 miles or 42 kilometers. An ultramarathon is technically anything over that and typically ranges up to 100 miles. A popular distance for women's racing events is 10 kilometers (6.2 miles — known as the mini-marathon).

phase. On the fourth, fifth, and sixth days of the pre-race period, the diet reverses to lean heavily on carbohydrates (any kind — from pasta to pastry). The theory is that the carbohydrate-loading phase allows the muscle tissues to absorb more glycogen than would have been possible without the depletion phase.

This diet is not for all runners — there are several disadvantages. First, low-glucose levels mean very low energy levels. By the end of the third day the dieter is likely to feel so fatigued that she is thoroughly discouraged about simple running, let alone racing. Second, because the high-protein phase of the first three days is lacking in roughage, it's quite common for a runner to be constipated by the time she shifts to the carbohydrate-loading phase. Third, it's argued that the depletion stage is associated with very small increases in the glycogen storage capacity, so that the slight benefit is more than offset by the negative effects. A popular modification of this diet emphasizes natural fruits and whole-grain products during the carbohydrate-loading phase, and avoids all processed "junk" foods, which are full of refined sugars and starches. (Be careful here: too much roughage and diarrhea will appear, instead of constipation.)

I think the modifications in a pre-race diet should be cautious ones. The fewer changes in your usual diet, the better you're likely to feel. If you're curious about any diet variations, check them out well in advance of the race. The best way to go to the starting line is with a gastrointestinal tract that is free of irritation and virtually empty. I try to eat on the light side and avoid large amounts of carbohydrates during the final three pre-race days. I also try to avoid consuming large amounts of dairy products (except yogurt, which is partially pre-digested). The sugar in milk — lactose — is readily converted into lactic acid, and an accumulation of lactic acid hampers racing effort tremendously. I skip the pre-race meal entirely because I normally train on an empty stomach and don't want to alter that pattern before a race. A number of runners I know simply eat two bananas, which are supremely digestible and rich in potassium — one of the body's essential electrolytes that can be lost in sweat during a race.

If the race you'll be running is scheduled for midday in a warm-weather month, do some of your pre-race training at that time of day. Get used to the heat, and treat hot weather with respect. Few other things are as potentially dangerous to a runner.

Fluid intake is crucial in hot-weather running to prevent serious dehydration. The combination of heat and humidity prevents the body's sweating mechanism from working efficiently to keep the body from overheating. Hot temperatures cause profuse sweating, but high humidity prevents evaporation, without which there is no heat loss. Therefore, the runner's internal body temperature rises while she continues to lose water and electrolytes in sweat. This can cause dizziness, cramps, nausea, and diarrhea; and it's possible for the afflicted runner to lapse into heat exhaustion or even heat stroke. The problem is an insidious one — it can affect an experienced runner as well as the novice — and the symptoms can make the runner feel "wiped out" and disoriented. Every racer must monitor herself as she goes along, staying alert for these early warning signs that the temperature regulation and water balance systems are going haywire. If any of these signs appear, you'll have to revise your expected finishing time and slow your pace accordingly (while replenishing fluids).

Any race over three miles long should have an aid station on the route where water (at least) and an electrolyte-replacement beverage (preferably) are available for the runners. Plan one or two trial runs of the race distance, stashing away a thermos of Gatorade, ERG, or water at several points along your route. That way you can gauge your body's fluid needs, get it accustomed to drinking on the run, and find out how well you tolerate the various beverages. If the electrolyte drinks give you intestinal problems, dilute them or stick to water — replacing fluid is more important than replacing electrolytes.

Consider what you'll wear in the race. Avoid anything brand-new, particularly shoes. *Never* race in shoes that haven't been broken in. If you'll be wearing a sweat shirt or jacket over your shorts to the starting line, be sure to pin your number to the bottom layer of clothing. That way your number won't be left behind with the spouse or friend holding the sweat shirt. If you're making a strong racing effort, dress more lightly than you would for a normal, slower-paced run.

The only thing you can't test beforehand is the extent of your pre-race nervousness. Many runners try to offset this by standing around in small groups and chatting aimlessly. I think it's better to work out the tension physically, rather than talking it through. I like to leave ample time between check-in and race-time, and I use it for:

- a trip to the bathroom.
- some thorough yoga-type stretching combined with relaxed deep breathing. I always include a chest-expansion exercise which opens up the rib cage so you can fill your lungs with air the minute the race begins. Do this one immediately before the actual start (see rib-cage stretch photograph, page 56). Use a sidewalk bench, a low fence padded with a sweat shirt, or almost anything that will support your lower back and permit you to arch over backward as in a backbend. Raise your arms above your head and let head and arms hang loosely, allowing grav-

ity to exert a substantial stretch on your rib cage. Do some deep breathing at the same time to enhance the stretch by inflating the lungs fully.

- some light running to shift the heart and lungs into gear before racing.
- a good long drink.
- another trip to the bathroom.

Even after going through your own personal ritual, you may still have a queasy feeling at the start of a race. This is partly because the body is gearing itself for strenuous activity and adrenalin is pouring into the bloodstream. What generally dispels the "butterflies" is the running itself. It's amazing how the starting gun helps all qualms disappear.

## Running the New York City Marathon

Two years after my first race I took off with thousands of other runners who were making their way across the Verrazano-Narrows Bridge as they began the October 1978 New York City Marathon. By this time I had considerably more experience — but it was *running* experience, not *racing* experience. I'd run a grand total of seven races in the interim (including the Boston and New York City Marathons in 1977) — not exactly a heavy racing schedule.

I had a lot of mixed feelings about New York '78. A stress fracture and a pulled Achilles tendon had mandated a three-month layoff that spring (during which I'd biked rather than run), so all the prudent admonitions were drumming in my brain. Be sensible about this race, they insisted. Don't risk injury and jeopardize running every day for the sake of a single race. I was willing to listen — injuries and layoffs are not exactly terrific.

There were other pressures too. Fred Lebow, the president of the New York Road Runners Club (and the moving force behind the marathon) had arranged for Mayor Edward Koch to sign me up as the 1978 marathon's first female entrant. That had already taken place at City Hall in July, and the ceremony had prompted a call from CBS News, who wanted to cover the race from a different point of view — through the experience of someone *not* in the lead pack with the elite runners. CBS said they just needed me to finish the marathon — time wasn't important. All this reinforced my conservative instincts. With the camera crews present, I thought I had to hold back and take it easy so I could finish in stand-up shape.

My most immediate worry, though, was a smoldering infection in a blister that had opened up in the arch of my foot — after being rubbed by the tape used to hold a metatarsal pad in place, said pad placed there to relieve a neuroma (a painful inflammation of the sensory nerve ending between the toes). I know that sounds almost comic, but running that way was no joke, and the injury bothered me from the first mile.

Interspersed with these concerns was a tiny seed of dissatisfaction. I'd run a 3:10 in the 1977 New York City Marathon — did I really want to make a poorer showing this year? Since I had started running again at the end of June I'd been putting in the miles — more than one hundred a week. But all my training had been LSD, with emphasis on *slow* and *long* — my pace seldom dipped under eight minutes a mile, which would come out to a 3:30 marathon. In September I ran two races to check whether my heel could take strenuous effort and to try to gauge what kind of marathon I might expect to run. The two races were the New York Road Runners Club First Annual Women's Half-Marathon in Central Park and the ten-mile Sri Chinmoy race in Greenwich. Both races served as a tease. Since I'd done the half-marathon in 1:25, could I break the 3-hour mark in this race? Of course I knew that you don't simply double time when you double distance, but the half-marathon made it plain that I could afford to slow down (losing as much as ten minutes) in the second half of the marathon and still be on target for three hours. The possibilities were intriguing — and part of me wanted to show CBS that the mother-housewife turned marathoner didn't have to slog her way through the 26 miles.

The week before the marathon had been bedlam. Jim was in California, where he'd been trying a case for six weeks, so my child-care duties were full-time. My foot was bothering me as the result of my one long pre-marathon run. (Twenty-two miles at a slow pace a week and a half before the race. Somehow I had to go through the motions of that long run to assure myself that I could manage the big race.) Then the CBS crew turned up at our home to follow me on some training runs. (I was wired for sound so that the birds and crickets *and* my breathing were recorded for background authenticity.) Later in the week Jim got back and my parents arrived to help with the children. Just in time — because the kids were more impish than usual.

On Sunday (marathon morning) the family contingent left for New York. My parents, my children, my cousin, *her* children, assorted friends, and Jim assembled at various places. Jim planned to wait at First Avenue in Manhattan, where he would join me for the last ten miles of the marathon. My cousin packed an enormous picnic lunch and led the clan to the Sheep Meadow in Central Park, where they would wait for the marathon to finish. I'd left much earlier than the rest of the group, traveling in a rented bus to the starting line in Staten Island with other local runners. The

CBS crew that waited for me there began filming as I stretched, jogged, and tried to ignore the camera. A military band played, I had a few mouthfuls of lukewarm coffee and long drinks of water, and then I followed the throng as it began to move up an incline toward the marathon start at the bridge's toll booth. Fifteen minutes later we were off, ambling forward in pretty disorderly fashion, and quickly packing the length of the bridge. The temperature was well into the 60s (it peaked just shy of 80 that day). I was glad I was dressed lightly in just nylon tank top and racing shorts, but the warmth of the day meant that fluids and pacing would figure importantly in the outcome of the race. The morning was bright and the view going over the bridge was spectacular — but our start was noisy because of all the helicopters buzzing overhead.

I was aware of the mile-long incline to the center of the bridge, but only because I watched the roadbed rise, crest, level off, then fall as we approached Brooklyn on the other side. My legs never felt the incline at all — there was too much adrenalin flowing for me to be aware of any effort. I did notice immediately, though, a small sharp twinge in the ball of my foot every time I landed, and I damned that neuroma.

Crowds lined the streets where we swung off the bridge into Brooklyn, but throughout the race they hardly registered. I stayed pretty much inside myself, concentrating on keeping my stride relaxed and smooth and my breathing regular and deep. Any outward attention was directed to the road — at the flow pattern of the runners — so I wouldn't be boxed in, or forced to take a too-wide turn. When I did look up to take in the larger view, it was to try to sight a landmark or an aid station up ahead.

The first marker was the digital clock at 5 miles. My racing experience is so limited that I still have difficulty in judging my pace, but when the digital clock flashed 31 minutes as I passed by, I was shocked. I'd never run 5 miles that fast before, and I still had 21 to go. I began to lecture myself to slow down. I wanted to be in respectable shape at the finish, not only because of the CBS cameras, but also because the children had seen me "done in" once before, and I didn't want to refresh that particular memory. We passed the Williamsburg Savings Bank — a conspicuous landmark — at 8 miles. Several miles later, when we were still wading through Brooklyn, my body began to complain. I slowed down — being careful not to cut back my breathing. Even though it was discouraging to let some of the field pass by me, I told myself that all those runners were probably headed toward times in the 2:40s, and that I had no business trying to keep up with them. Actually, this was only a brief slowdown and it probably saved the marathon for me.

We crossed the Pulaski Bridge into Queens halfway through the race, and the digital clock showed I was running well ahead of my half-marathon time the month before. The section through Queens was a series of right-angled turns — it coursed like a maze through streets filled with warehouses. When I saw the elevated structure ahead I realized we were approaching another bridge — the Queensborough this time. We were Manhattan-bound at last! The metal grating of the pedestrian walkway had been covered by a 3-foot wide strip of broadloom by an enterprising carpet company. The carpet was really too plush and gave no traction at all, but it felt wonderful under my sore foot. I recall glancing at my watch at this point. It was not quite 12:10 and I thought, "Not bad . . . an hour and twenty minutes left to cover the last ten miles." Then it struck me that in a half-hour or so the race would be over for champion Bill Rodgers and a few others like him.

Swinging down the bridge ramp, we were greeted with deafening roars by the crowd. Looping around under the bridge before turning to head up First Avenue, I hadn't gone far before spotting Jim. He fairly jumped out of the crowd at 64th Street and fell into stride beside me. We smiled, but didn't say much.

Now we were running between two solid walls of spectators and sometimes the passageway was so narrow that we were forced to hold the same pace as the runners right around us. It was impossible to set your own pace, impossible to ignore the wild cheering, and equally impossible to think of dropping out at that point. Those first miles in Manhattan are such a high that it takes a while to notice that First Avenue is basically an uphill climb. I knew I was making good time, but I was working harder now. I was also more aware of the pain in my foot. I caught myself bracing for it by tightening that left leg all the way up the back. It put a distinct hitch in my stride, and I hoped I wasn't noticeably limping. I tried to stay loose, to smooth out my stride, and I kept drinking water.

As 20 miles approached we veered into the Bronx. It seemed like a pointless detour at that stage, since we'd already been in Manhattan. There were 6.2 miles to go, and I knew they'd be the toughest. In the Bronx I encountered the one obstacle in the race — a foot-high curbstone at a pedestrian walkway. I'd almost fallen there the previous year, but now Jim reminded me of it as we approached. Running along 138th Street gave me a terrific boost: the spectators were particularly enthusiastic.

The last bridge brought us back into Manhattan. Fifth Avenue southbound was also uphill, especially the last few blocks before we entered the park at 102nd Street. I took another quick glance at my watch — it was one o'clock. I wondered vaguely if Rodgers had won again, then it hit me — with just three miles to go I might finish inside of three hours.

The crowds were huge now. I heard someone calling my name and saw several friends wildly jumping and waving. What a burst of energy *that* gave me! The course dipped out of the park to run along Central Park South before entering again at Columbus Circle, where it became an undulating ribbon of roadway — up and down, up and down. Every part of me was bent on finishing now — I couldn't allow myself a single wasted motion, breath, or stride. The runners struggled and the crowd matched that intensity with their cheers.

By this time my left leg was cramping badly, thanks to the neuroma. To counteract involuntarily tensing that leg, I found myself tensing my forearms instead. My fingers were outstretched, as if to draw the tension away from my leg and out through my fingertips. I'm sure it looked weird and I know it was inefficient — but it seemed to work. I managed to keep to a steady pace. I was aware of passing several other women runners in this loop through the park. I knew we were getting near the finish line from the din of the people massed on either side. Finally, I could see the finish banner up ahead. While Jim jumped ecstatically up and down, waving his arms overhead, I simply kept going in a straight line, my eyes focused on the finishing chutes. Then suddenly I found myself being directed toward the left-hand chute. I looked up at the digital clock at the finish line to catch the time — 2:54:33 — as I entered the chute. Jim followed me in and as we slowed down, he threw his arms around my shoulders. I turned toward him and we fell into an embrace that was duly recorded by the CBS cameras on the photobridge overhead.

We picked up some bottles of Perrier water at the end of the chute and kept walking — aimlessly at first — just to keep our muscles from cramping. Then the CBS producer led us over to the Sheep Meadow, where the rest of the family was spread out on the grass, with a picnic in full progress.

Our reunion was wonderful — much hugging and kissing and excited shouts from the kids. Breaking the 3-hour mark was deeply satisfying, but what made the '78 marathon so special was having my family there to share the experience with me — to be with my husband, children, and parents on such a happy day.

SIX

# RUNNING AND YOUR BODY

## *Running's Effect on the Marvelous Machine—Plus Stress Points, No-no's, and Injuries*

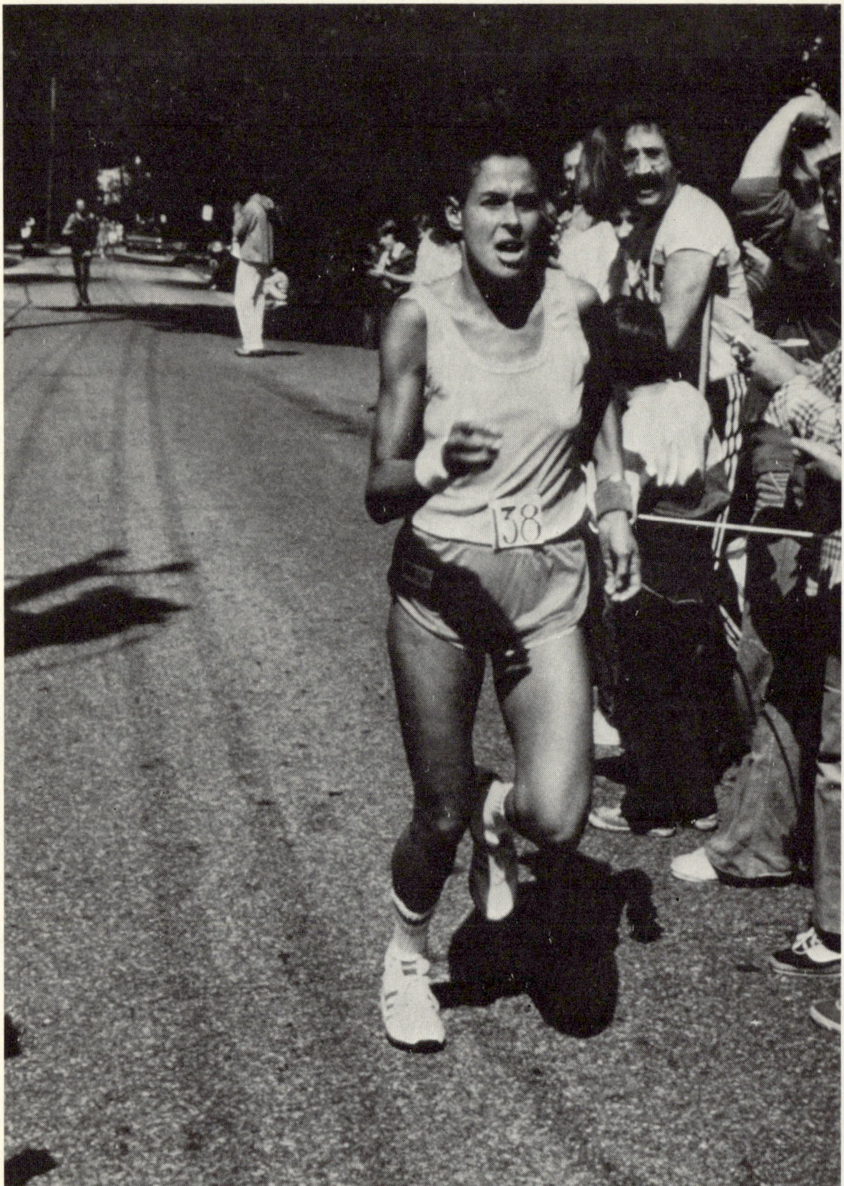

Pushing toward the finish — the Sri Chinmoy 10-miler, September 1978. *Lloyd Hart*

Mary Dono is a Westchester, New York, mother of four (two girls, 10 and 9, and 2-year-old twin boys) who is also a registered nurse. She began running nine years ago, when there were few women runners, and it took her a long time to surmount what she now calls "my embarrassment about how I looked." She also found herself struggling with the "beginner's syndrome" in running — a combination of breathlessness, side-stitches, and leg pains in muscles and tendons.

"My first runs were in the driveway of the local high school," she says. "I did very little at first — a mile of walk-run-walk. Then I went out on the road and just ran the mile. The distance increased very gradually, but it took me two months to feel comfortable. After 6 or 7 weeks, I began experiencing more good days than bad — more days when I 'felt loose' and had good control of my running. The heavy breathing was the first to go. I did yoga stretching at home which helped my legs, so I felt lighter on my feet. And as I felt better physically, my mental attitude improved too. The psychological ingredients blended with the physical to make my running really pleasurable for me."

Mary's experience mirrors that of many novice runners.

They begin with heart hammering, lungs feeling as though they might burst, pains in the legs, and feelings of general stress. These symptoms appear because the new runner is taxing the ability of the heart and lungs to deliver oxygen to the working muscles — primarily the legs. As the heart-lung machine improves its efficiency, the aerobic capacity increases, along with the ease in handling the workout. This conditioning effect is achieved by repeated exercise-induced elevation of the pulse rate and the rate of breathing. No conditioning is possible without some hard work — you have to stress the organs in order to get the conditioning effect. The key to reasonable progress is a program that delivers the stress in small increments. Get comfortable with the length of a particular run before you increase your distance. At these beginning stages, *you cannot proceed too slowly,* because your body is trying to integrate many changes.

## The CVR Training Effect

Training has a pronounced effect on cardiac function: the heart muscle increases in size and its pumping action improves, enabling it to eject a larger volume of blood with each stroke. This means that the heart doesn't have to beat so frequently to maintain the same volume of blood in circulation — and this change is reflected in the resting heart rate. The average resting heart rate for U.S. men is 72 beats per minute, for women it's often in the 80s. For trained athletes of either sex, resting pulse rates in the 40s and 50s are not unusual. (Tennis champion Bjorn Borg has a resting pulse rate in the 30s!)

Training also has a definite impact on pulmonary function: the lungs inflate more fully (with the cooperation of the muscles of the chest, stomach, and diaphragm), so that more air is inhaled with each breath. At the same time the lungs improve their efficiency in extracting more oxygen from the air they inhale and delivering that oxygen to the bloodstream — making more oxygen available to the tissues. These changes in the cardiovascular and respiratory (CVR) systems are lumped together in the term "CVR training effect."

How does exercise bring about these beneficial changes? When you exercise your body, your muscles (especially the large motor muscles) are doing the work. These muscles — like the parts of any good machine — need fuel to do the job. The fuels come from the carbohydrates, fats, and proteins in the foods you eat — but the muscles also need large amounts of oxygen in order to burn the foods efficiently and extract maximum energy. The muscles, therefore, need more oxygen delivered to them at a rapid rate so they can keep on working.* To do this, the body turns to its own oxygen-delivery system (the coordinated action of the heart, blood vessels, and lungs) to rush more oxygen to the tissues. This is why the heart and lungs are the first to feel the effects of running — and the marvel of their adaptability is that they respond so dramatically to the physical effort.

## The Musculoskeletal System

Less obvious at the start than your hammering heart and bursting lungs are the adaptive changes that occur in your musculoskeletal system when you work your body strenuously. These effects are more subtle, but sooner or later they begin to emerge. You'll notice a reshaping of certain areas

* An endurance exercise such as LSD running is a classic example of an aerobic exercise because the heart-lung machine is able to deliver ample oxygen to sustain the activity. In contrast, an anaerobic exercise (such as sprinting) is one in which you're working at a rate that outstrips the body's ability to supply enough oxygen to sustain the activity.

of the body — a streamlining of the hips and thighs, less general fleshiness with sharper muscle definition. These are encouraging signs that the muscles are "firming up" in training, and that your running is working off the kind of fat (called "intramuscular") that is marbled throughout the muscle tissue. The muscles appear leaner — especially if there has been a general loss of weight and the muscles are no longer blanketed by a layer of subcutaneous (under-the-skin) fat.

It's not only the muscle tissue that strengthens with the repeated contractions of regular endurance exercise. Tendons also become thicker and stronger, and — amazingly — the long bones of the legs become stronger and their circumference increases (as more calcium is deposited). So much for the popular notion that bones are brittle, static structures once growth is complete!

## The Stress-Overload Principle

The common pitfall of the new runner is to use these positive signs of increasing fitness to train much harder — often *too* hard. Every runner should train with the awareness that the human body can be pushed too far. This marvelous machine at our command is adaptable — within limits. There's real merit in the phrase "Train, don't strain!"

Any conditioning program — from running to weightlifting — works on the stress-overload principle: the body responds to unusual stress by making the necessary adaptation so that it can handle that same stress the next time. The body adjusts if the appropriate conditions are met. First, the increase in stress must be within reasonable boundaries. Excess stress produces strain — if continued it can weaken the body. Second, whenever new stress is imposed, adequate time must be allowed for the body to complete both phases of the adaptive process — recovery and strengthening. If the stress is repeated too soon (or worse, if it's increased) conditioning will not improve, it will deteriorate.

Certain training guidelines emphasize these principles — an obvious example is the "hard-easy" rule, upon which a good program for building up your weekly mileage would rely. By this principle if you wanted to increase your base mileage from 30 to 33, your schedule would be:

Week 1 — 30 miles
Week 2 — 33 miles
Week 3 — 30 miles
Week 4 — 33 miles (at this point you may stay with increased mileage)

This one step forward–one back–another step forward approach may seem overly cautious, but it provides an extra margin of safety against the kind of unrelieved stress that accompanies insufficient recovery time. This seesaw routine also insures that weekly mileage totals don't increase too fast. (The best plan for mileage buildup is no more than 5 miles per week or 10 per cent of your weekly average, whichever is less.) The extra time this approach requires is far less than the time spent in sitting out overstress injuries. It's particularly unwise to schedule strenuous interval workouts several days in a row.

Vary your workouts as much as possible, mixing pace and style, switching surfaces and terrain frequently. This kind of training diversity promotes better all-round musculoskeletal adaptation, and lessens the risks of serious overuse injuries. David Propp says, "The more versatile a runner is, the more efficient and graceful she's likely to be . . . and the less likely she is to be injured."

Generally, a runner's conditioning process seems to encounter fewer hitches in CVR adaptation than in the musculoskeletal adjustment. For average runners (those with no cardiac abnormalities) the musculoskeletal system is the more delicate — and should be favored. Dr. Gary Gallo, an orthopedic surgeon who specializes in sports medicine, taught me this lesson one day when I sat in his examining room, ruefully eyeing a swollen Achilles tendon. Dr. Gallo explained that the cardiovascular system has a built-in safety mechanism. When the heart is pushed to its maximum, you can't get it to beat any faster, no matter how much additional work you give it. Unfortunately, there's no such safety device for the musculoskeletal system. Muscles, tendons, and bones are all vulnerable when increasing stress is applied — they keep trying to cope with the additional work, but give *out* before they give *in*.

## Stresses, Injuries, and No-No's

With the huge increase in numbers of new runners (more and more of them women) orthopedists now see as many stress fractures from roadrunning as regular fractures from skiing, and podiatrists may treat as many running injuries as ordinary bunions. Sports medicine is no longer restricted to team physicians who are treating professional athletes.

Don't let this alarm you. Dr. Gallo's experience has been that it's the new runner who most often comes in to see him. Seasoned runners become quite expert at dealing with minor injuries and manage to stay out of his office. Dr. Gallo also feels that — in the realm of athletic injuries — those afflicting runners are relatively mild. That view is supported by Dr. Robert Brown, a psychiatrist at the University of Virginia and a consultant with the National Institute of Mental Health, who wryly comments that it's better to be visiting the orthopedist than the cardiologist or internist. "The ravages of activity," Dr. Brown says, "are clearly preferable to the ravages of inactivity."

Still it may not console the injured runner to know that

she's suffering from what Dr. George Sheehan calls a "disease of excellence." An injury that may not be severe from an orthopedic standpoint may seem critical to the runner who has to endure it. From the runner's point of view, any injury that forces her to quit running — even temporarily — is serious. And that's where most of the problems crop up. By refusing to deal realistically with an injury (or an injury-in-the-making), a runner can vastly complicate her condition.

Except in the case of injuries due to accidental trauma (rare in running compared to the acute injuries suffered in skiing or contact sports), the onset of most running injuries is gradual. It's the repetitive action of running — the use of muscles, tendons, ligaments, bones, and joints in the same way over and over again — that causes most running injuries. The chronic conditions that may result are described as the "overuse syndrome." In short, wear and tear are responsible, but not every runner reacts to the same degree — some log an incredible number of miles without any problems whatever. To make her injury-prone, the runner's overuse factor must be joined by a weak link somewhere in her musculoskeletal system. This can be anything from a muscular imbalance (overdeveloped muscles along the back of the leg and underdeveloped muscles along the front) to some biomechanical deviation from the normal structure in the foot, ankle, knee joint, or hip. How far and how fast you can run while remaining injury-free is directly related to the soundness of your musculoskeletal system.

## Pain — The Prime Body Signal

Obviously you can't run to the doctor with every minor pain, but there *is* a middle ground between hypochondria and masochistic neglect. Finding it is not simple. It's hard to distinguish the point at which previously random aches and pains merge and intensify, indicating possible injury. Even experienced runners find this hard to do — they may be better able to "read" their bodies, but they're also better at tuning out pain. Dr. William P. Morgan, professor of physical education and director of the Sport Psychology Laboratory at the University of Wisconsin, believes that dissociating from pain is a potentially dangerous practice, especially during races. "Runners are urged to pay attention to the signals from their bodies," Dr. Morgan says. "Pain should be viewed as a positive sensation, and the runner should learn to respond to it appropriately."

The sensible approach is to become more sophisticated about pain. It's hardly a welcome friend, but it's not an enemy either. Pain is instructive, and the prudent runner respects it. She soon recognizes different kinds of pain and understands their meaning.

The most common kind of running pain is the ache of stiff muscles at the very beginning of a run. This most often occurs when you haven't stretched properly before the workout. If this happens, take a few minutes more with your stretching routine or break into your run very gradually. (You can also stop and stretch again along the way.) Sometimes there's a generalized soreness in the legs which feels like a carry-over from the previous day's run. In this case, go easy — and shorten your workout if it doesn't ease up.

If you're aware of the problem area, check it carefully before you go out to run. Slowly move, bend, and stretch it, testing the limits of flexibility and the range of pain; if the problem is simply muscle tightness, you may succeed in working out the tension. If you can't release it completely, it's probably still all right to run. Choose level ground, don't try for speed, and monitor the spot en route. Stop at frequent intervals to stretch, and shorten your workout if the pain or stiffness worsens. Any strain severe enough to force you to change your running style (stride, foot-plant, etc.) can cause a second injury worse than the first.

Self-diagnosis is a tricky business, but with practice every runner can develop a keen alertness to her body's signals. The most adept runners develop such sensitive feedback systems that they can respond to the first symptoms before stress turns into distress. David Propp, for instance, averages 25 miles a day and remains virtually injury-free. His success is due to his supple frame, the variety and flexibility of his training habits, and the sophisticated level of body awareness he has developed. Body awareness doesn't develop automatically as the running proceeds — it requires conscious effort. The sharp and intuitive runner is better able to recognize, evaluate, and often prevent many of the ailments that follow.

*Runner's Knee*

The medical term for "runner's knee" is *chondromalacia patella,* which means a softening of the undersurface of the kneecap (patella). The patella normally rides in a groove on the femur (thighbone), but stress may cause the patella to veer from the groove, resulting in excessive rotation of the knee at footstrike. When this happens, abnormal softening and wear occur — accompanied by pain, stiffness, and swelling. The stresses that cause chondromalacia are often biomechanical — defects of the hips, knees, and feet. Morton's Foot (a condition in which the first toe is shorter than the second) is sometimes the culprit. Since the first toe usually absorbs most of the impact when the foot hits the turf, knee, leg, heel, and back problems result when the first toe is unstable. The condition may be helped by inserts like Dr. Scholl's flexo pads, which provide arch support and incorporate a metatarsal pad. If these don't provide relief, many runners resort to orthotics, custom-made inserts (rigid or semiflexible) that are fitted by a podiatrist, who takes a plaster mold of the foot.

Knee pain, on the other hand, also may be due to faulty development of the quadriceps (front thigh) muscle, so that it pulls unevenly on the knee cap, causing it to slide off its groove. Exercises that strengthen the quadriceps help to normalize knee function. The simplest and most effective of these exercises involves sitting on a table or bench high enough to allow the legs to hang free. Suspend an old handbag (with a wide, soft strap) filled with children's blocks or sand (this is more comfortable than the usually prescribed paint can) across the instep of the foot and then raise the lower leg, extending it straight out. Hold this position for a slow count of ten, before lowering the leg again. Repeat five times with each leg. The weight can gradually be increased as the quadriceps strengthen.

When women experience knee problems they should first consider the quadriceps muscles as the source of the trouble, since weak quadriceps are more common in unconditioned females. Ligaments that support the knee joint, either at the inside or outside of the knee, are also subject to strain. Here biomechanical deviations may not be the only problem. Shoes that are worn down excessively or even the slant of the road can cause strain. When you have pain, always check your shoes first. Then check the road surface to see whether it slopes down toward the affected leg. If this is the case, run on level ground, reverse direction, or switch to the other side of the road.

### *Ankle Problems*

*Achilles Tendinitis.* The Achilles tendon is a thin cord that connects the heel bone with the calf muscle, and Achilles tendinitis is an inflammation of that tendon. The heel area can become swollen and painful, making running, or even walking, very difficult. The condition can be partially genetic; many people are born with short Achilles tendons that don't tolerate much stress. It's more usually caused, however, by tight calf muscles that put too much strain on the tendon. Good ways to prevent Achilles tendinitis are these:

- Do thorough warm-ups, including stretching exercises for the calves (especially the wall pushup mentioned on page 52).
- Wear shoes with good heel supports, or add heel lifts.
- Avoid both too much speed and too many hills in your workouts.

If you develop Achilles tendinitis and suspect you have more than a simple inflammation, don't run. A raspy, grating feeling along the tendon means friction between the tendon sheath and the tendon itself and may indicate you are tearing tendon fibers. Apply ice packs to the tendon, elevate the leg, and *rest*. If there's no improvement, see a doctor.

*Sprains*. Dr. Gallo believes that the incidence of sprained ankles is far rarer in running than in other physical activities, since a runner's ankles are strengthened by the sport. "From a layman's point of view," he says, "running is a safe activity and serious injuries are rare. Most runners are stronger, more agile, and more conscious of taking care of themselves." However, it's possible to plant your foot in an unsuspected hole. If you suffer a sprain, see a doctor.

### *Foot Problems*

*Heel Bruises*. A heel bruise is a rather common inflammation suffered by long-distance runners and is caused by the amount of pounding that the runner's foot must bear. Heel cups and ice packs help with these inflammations — and so does running on grass instead of on hard surfaces. (Heel cups can be found where your running shoes are sold.)

*Plantar Fasciitis.* The plantar fascia is the connective tissue that runs the length of the sole. As the foot pounds on the run, the arch is flattened and lengthened, and the plantar fascia is stretched. This can result in tears in the fascia where it attaches to the heel bone. Pain in the heel is the principle symptom, and arch supports with heel cups or a very well-cushioned shoe provide the relief.

*Heel Spurs.* Heel spurs may occur either on the bottom of the heel where the plantar fascia and muscles join the heel bone, or on the back of the heel where the Achilles tendon attaches to the heel. Both types are identified by the build-up of a "bony bump" (the characteristic spur), but their causes are distinctly different. Heel spurs that develop on the bottom of the heel are generally due to strains of the plantar fascia and are far less common in runners than spurs on the back of the heel. The back-of-the-heel spur is often caused by an overly tight Achilles tendon, and results in the painful "runner's bump" that develops at the base of the heel cord (Achilles) where it attaches to the heel bone. A shoe that does not fit properly in the heel area may also cause this condition. If the heel counter is too snug, or rises too high, it may irritate the base of the Achilles tendon. If the heel counter is too loose, friction and rubbing of the heel against the shoe may produce the same condition. If the heel bone itself is biomechanically unstable, it may roll too much inside the shoe. When the cause of a spur is a true, tight Achilles tendon, then the tendon should be thoroughly stretched by exercises such as the wall pushup. The surrounding musculature may also be strengthened with toe lifts — rising up on the ball of the foot and holding for a brief count before lowering again. If your running shoes have caused or aggravated the condition, then look for a shoe with a lower, snugger, or wider heel counter depending on the fit problem. A heel lift that provides added height also helps relieve the strain on a tight Achilles tendon.

*Forefoot Neuroma.* Many runners suffer from a general pain along the ball of the foot. This is most often due to the fact that the protective fat pad on the bottom of the foot gets pushed up under the toe area in the course of a run, allowing the ligaments and the heads of the metatarsal bones to bear the brunt of the running impact. This condition is called "plantar metatarsalgia" and is helped by a shoe that is heavily cushioned in the forefoot area.

Plantar metatarsalgia may also be accompanied by damage to the interdigital nerves, which run between the toes. Stress to the nerve tissue can cause traumatic neuroma, most commonly between the third and fourth toes. During a run the neuroma can cause a sharp, shooting pain in this area, which will also feel tender to the touch. A highly padded shoe that is fitted with a cushioned insole should help alleviate this condition.

### *Shin Splints*

Shin splints are indicated by the presence of a deep, diffuse, but persistent pain along the front of the shin bone, or along its side. They are primarily due to overstressed or inflamed muscles and tendons and are caused by many factors — including hard-surface jolts, inadequate warm-ups, running on the toes, or running in shoes that are worn thin. If you develop shin splints, avoid running on pavement, sidewalk, or hills. Don't run on your toes, either. Wear thickly cushioned shoes with a good heel lift, and heavy socks as well. If this doesn't help, stop running and try ice, rest, elevation, and this excellent exercise: use a weighted handbag suspended across the instep of your foot (as with the quadriceps exercise), but flex the foot *only* (do not raise your leg), pointing toes up toward the knee.

*Stress Fractures*

Stress fractures can appear anywhere — in the metatarsal bones of the foot, in the heel, the lower leg, or even the thigh and hip — but they most often occur in the metatarsals and the lower leg bones (tibia and fibula). A West Point survey of a cadet training program indicates that women may be more vulnerable to stress fractures than men. There were 102 women and 1228 men in the test group, and stress fractures occurred in 10 of the women and 12 of the men — a female-to-male ratio of 12 to 1.

The best treatment for stress fracture is rest — which was the therapy prescribed for me when I suffered a stress fracture of the right fibula (a few inches up from the ankle bone). I'd noticed tenderness and swelling around the ankle and thought I'd been bruised. Somehow I didn't think of it as a running injury and simply continued to work out, though the pain and swelling increased. Returning one Saturday morning from an 11-mile run, I found I couldn't walk. Chastened, I spent all the next day using ice, rest, and elevation (the runner's IRE). On Monday morning I presented myself to the doctor. An extended rest period followed, during which I swam for exercise.

*Blisters*

Since I am plagued with blisters, I envy runners who simply put on their shoes and shoot out the door. I spend a lot of good running time on preventive care — dressing, padding, and protecting blisters — before I start on my workout. The problem with blisters is that they're not serious enough to keep you off your feet, but *do* require healing time. Most runners choose to keep on running (I'm one of these), and aggravate the blisters with each workout. The operative question is: how do you prevent a simple blister from escalating into an infection?

If the blister is new, you might try applying ice right away. This may help to reabsorb some fluid — at any rate, the blister won't "puff up" so much. If it's not too sore, avoid puncturing it. Dr. Giannone recommends applying petroleum jelly to ease friction and then wrapping the blister with lamb's wool and tape, or covering it with a Band-Aid. If the blister is quite painful or filled with fluid, flame a needle (or use Merthiolate or Betadine to disinfect it — alcohol is not as good) and prick the blister open, being careful to evacuate all the fluid. Then apply an antibiotic ointment (such as Bacitracin) before you cover it with a Band-Aid. Remember, if you decide to open the blister, it's *imperative* to keep it clean. If you're running on a blister, don't keep using the shoes that caused it in the first place. Be aware that the insides of your shoes and socks provide the perfect moist environment for bacteria. Proper hygiene means changing bandages before you run, soaking the area immediately afterward, and then applying a clean dressing. Except when you're soaking it, keep the blister dry, clean, and covered.

Whether you decide to puncture the blister or leave it alone, you'll want to protect it from further pressure if it's in a weight-bearing area. To do this, pad the area immediately around the blister with adhesive mole-foam or moleskin. Dr. Giannone stresses that it's important *not* to constrict the area by applying a "donut" that completely encircles the blister — leave one side open. In severe cases when this method doesn't give enough protection, I've used double layers of adhesive mole-foam and superimposed a "donut" on top of a "U-shape." Change the mole-foam if it gets too soggy from running or bathing.

Once the blister is completely healed or reabsorbed, you might try toughening the area by applying tincture of benzoin (let it dry after each application). This helps the skin resist further blistering. When you decide it's time to dispense with the adhesive bandage, apply a dab of petroleum jelly as a safety measure. A light coating of petroleum jelly is a good idea, anyhow, especially around toes, heels, or anywhere a callous indicates friction.

An alternative to the Band-Aid/ointment method is to wrap the toes (or dress the area) in gauze and saturate with Betadine. Reapply the Betadine several times a day and replace gauze at least daily. This dries out the blistered skin and wards off infection. If in spite of your best efforts, infection does set in, soak the foot for 20 minutes in warm salt water as often as you can during the day. Keep the infected area dry and covered at all other times. (Don't leave it uncovered overnight until all signs of infection are gone.)

*Toenails*

Blackened toenails ("runner's toes") are common among distance runners. The discoloration is due to bleeding under the nail plate and is caused by pressure on the nail during the running; what forms as a result is a blood blister or "hematoma." A few simple precautions may help you avoid runner's toes. First, keep your toenails short, smooth, and well-trimmed. Check your running shoes as well; they should fit snugly enough across the vamp to prevent excessive slippage toward the toes, there should be adequate room in the toe box, and the shoe should flex easily across the ball of the foot.

Despite all this, you may return from a run and notice a darkened toenail. Sometimes the fluid reabsorbs and the discoloration disappears by itself, but usually remedial steps must be taken. If there is swelling and pain and the nail plate is elevated, the trapped fluid must be released. The most frequently recommended way to do this is to puncture the nail plate by applying momentary pressure with a paper clip that has been straightened and sterilized with a flame. (This is a *painless* method — there are no nerves in the nail.) Personally, I prefer to release the pressure with a sterilized needle through the skin (where it joins the top of the nailplate), just as one would an ordinary blister. Either way, the damaged nail plate should be left in place for protection until a new nail has formed underneath. It is essential to keep the under-nail area clean and free of infection by frequent warm-water soaks. Between soaks — and this is crucial — a thin strand of sterile cotton saturated with alcohol or Betadine should be wedged under the upper edge of the nail and anchored around the corners. Secure the dressing in place with tape or an adhesive bandage.

## Consult Your Running Log

A good running log should not only have details like day, time, and distance, but should also list the kind of shoes you wore and the particulars of your course (terrain, underfoot surface, and departures from the route). If you keep a faithful record in the log, it can be an invaluable aid in figuring out what factors in the preceding week's run might have contributed to an injury.

## Racing Pain

If you elect to race and do train hard for it (with interval workouts, hill work, and increased speed) you should be prepared to face pain. The pain will be of a totally different order than those novice twinges and aches. Normally, long slow distance running (increased in easy, gradual stages) presents no great problems of discomfort. Its beauty is that *you* control the degree of effort and can minimize body strain.

But pitting yourself against pain — and overcoming it to accomplish your goal — is an integral part of the challenge of racing. The more you strive to realize your potential, the more you try for maximum performance — the more pain you'll encounter. In some running circles the subject of racing pain has been unfortunately glossed over with tidy euphemisms like "stress" and "unpleasant sensations." An effort is made to tiptoe around the subject, as in natural childbirth classes, where one speaks of "labor contractions" instead of "labor pains." There are some advantages to this approach — it reduces apprehension and raises positive expectations in running as in childbirth. However, the realistic runner knows that some degree of pain is one ingredient of a strenuous racing effort — and she makes emotional provision for that fact.

Citing Grantly Dick-Read's *Childbirth Without Fear,** George Sheehan comments, "What else in the course of everyday human experience can compare with a marathon but childbirth?" For all runners who are mothers, the analogy is apt. I've spoken to many women who have compared the two experiences, and the similarities go deeper than the common element of pain (compounded by fear of the unknown). When defining the impact of a marathon, these women referred to the birth experience in order to convey the singular and meaningful qualities of the race. Katie Baxter says, "I remember crossing the finish line in my first

* Dr. Dick-Read is universally regarded as the "godfather" of the modern natural childbirth movement. His book was the first to raise women's consciousness about the fact that they were being robbed of the birth experience.

marathon and thinking to myself that I hadn't been this happy since I gave birth. I had such a feeling of elation . . . such a sense of accomplishment and pride in myself."

Both the birth experience and marathon running impose a unique and rigorous discipline. Once you begin them they may take you to a place deep inside yourself — alternately stretching time or telescoping it, and conferring a primal sense of power. For the woman whose chances for physical self-expression have been culturally limited, both the marathon and childbirth provide confirmation of one fact: her body works. She doesn't need to win the race — or even run distinctively — to prove that point. Just reaching the finishing line proves she has great reserves of strength and stamina.

The day after I ran my first marathon — when I was still overwhelmed by the experience — I went to visit my cousin Melissa Hommer and her infant daughter. (I must say here that Melissa is no ordinary cousin. She is also a friend and sister who has "mothered" both me and my children when we needed her.) When I arrived Melissa asked the standard question, "What was it like?" I smiled and gave her an answer we both could understand. "It's hard work," I said, "the closest damn thing to giving birth . . . except that there's no baby at the end of it."

SEVEN

# RUNNING, MENSTRUATION, AND PREGNANCY

## *The Female Cycle and the Runner's Life*

I've often thought that women are particularly attuned to the rhythms of running because the steady beat of the physical workout prompts instinctive reference to the female cycle. While new awareness of our bodies has fostered healthy and practical attitudes about their function, certain elemental influences remain. The most powerful of these is the central fact that, for half her life, a woman's reproductive impulse beats in hormonal counterpoint to all her other efforts. The woman runner may find herself in particular rapport with these biological rhythms. She is functioning in a body made healthy by exercise and so is better able to cope with her menstrual periods and the hard work of bearing a child.

## Running and Your Menstrual Period

The myth that participation in strenuous sports can seriously disrupt a woman's reproductive cycle is one that has persisted far into the twentieth century. In 1963, two young women who ran illegally in California's Western Hemisphere Marathon were reprimanded by female AAU officials and bluntly told that racing would impair their ability to have children. More recently, a *Time* magazine cover story (June 1978) claimed that 45 per cent of women who ran over 65 miles per week experience menstrual irregularities. Unfortunately the story didn't say what percentage of women in a *nonrunning* population would also have menstrual problems — or whether the runners had the irregularities before they *ever started to run* (see Figure 2, Basal Body Temperature Chart, in the Appendix). Dr. Mona Shangold, assistant professor of obstetrics and gynecology at the Albert Einstein College of Medicine (and a marathon runner herself) believes that "*Most* women experience menstrual irregularities from time to time, and these are caused by many factors ranging from emotional stress to the common cold.

"A woman who is involved in a strenuous training program is not just exercising — she's involved in all kinds of pressures including the anxieties of competition. If she is incorporating 50 miles a week into an already busy schedule, she is probably contending with a tremendous amount of anxiety in merely carrying out all of her responsibilities. Such anxiety alone would prompt irregularities. My own theory is that women who develop amenorrhea [absence of the menstrual period] as runners or athletes have a heavier component of stress in their lives, and that this stress plays a larger role than heavy exercise in any menstrual irregularities that are present."

Any interruption of the menstrual cycle should concern runners of child-bearing age. (I'm annoyed with male physicians who suggest that lighter, fewer, or even absent periods are a welcome phenomenon.) Pinpointing the cause of a menstrual interruption is often tricky, though, since the regulation of the menstrual cycle and the process of ovulation depend on a precise shifting of the glandular gears.

As explained by Dr. Shangold, the initial impulse does not originate in the reproductive glands, but in the hypothalamus (located in the base of the brain) which secretes a releasing hormone (called $G_nRH$ — gonadotropin releasing hormone). This hormone, in turn, causes the pituitary gland to produce the hormones called FSH (follicle-stimulating hormone) and LH (luteinizing hormone). FSH and LH act on the ovaries, directing the complex sequence of events that governs the menstrual cycle. This influence does not simply go in one direction — from hypothalamus to pituitary to the ovaries; subtle positive and negative feedback systems are involved at each level. This "hypothalamic-pituitary-ovarian axis" is affected by its own internal processes and also by external influences, including the higher brain centers where anxiety and environmental factors are registered. As Dr. Shangold points out, "It's impossible to separate the influence of your external environment from your endocrine system. Considering the delicate balance required to effect this sophisticated program, it is much more surprising that women ever ovulate and menstruate regularly than that they do not."

If a woman runner is experiencing amenorrhea even though she may be unfazed by competition and free of serious stress, the reason may simply be a pronounced loss of body weight — and particularly body fat. Normal untrained women range from 25 to 30 per cent body fat; trained women runners may average 15 per cent or less. A certain minimum percentage of body fat is believed to be required for the onset of menstruation at puberty (17 per cent, according to one study) and for the maintenance of the cycle in women over 18 years (about 22 per cent). The correlation between low body fat and infrequency or cessation of the menstrual period is not absolutely clear-cut. Many women with less body fat have normal and regular periods, while some obese women do not ovulate at all. However, the woman runner whose training has made her thin should consider weight loss as a possible cause if her periods become irregular.

The sensible runner's rule is: if in doubt, see a doctor. Mona Shangold says, "The menstrual interval is defined as the number of days from the beginning of one period to the beginning of the next period. I consider a normal menstrual interval to be between 25 and 32 days. If a woman's menstrual interval is between 20 and 60 days, she doesn't need to do anything unless she's trying to become pregnant and is having difficulty doing so, in which case she should consult a specialist. If her menstrual interval is less than 20 days or more than 60 days, she should see a gynecologic endocrinologist. She should also seek attention if she bleeds between periods or has a breast discharge. In general, if her periods were regular before and have become irregular since she began running, she ought to be checked."

### *Dysmenorrhea*

There are a few dissenting opinions, but most sports-medical authorities agree that athletic participation helps alleviate such symptoms as cramps, nausea, headache, bloating, and depression that group under the umbrella-term "dysmenorrhea" (difficult or painful menstruation). Except for swimmers, who are reported to have the highest incidence of menstrual complaints, athletically active women have far fewer menstrual (and premenstrual) symptoms than their more sedentary counterparts.

If you *are* one of those women who experience some degree of menstrual discomfort, remember that there's no rule that says you have to run every day. On the other hand, these problems can often be helped by something as simple as aspirin.* Dr. Shangold recommends that a woman begin taking aspirin just before she expects her pain — two tablets every four hours. She can continue this right through the difficult part of her cycle, as long as she shows no sign of toxicity. (Ringing in the ears is the first sign of aspirin toxicity.) Someone who cannot anticipate the pain can take three aspirins when it starts and then two tablets every four hours. Aspirin is also helpful in relieving some of the side effects of intrauterine devices. IUD-wearers who experience cramps and heavy bleeding during their periods may not want to run on those days. Because heavy bleeding can cause iron loss, Dr. Shangold recommends that every woman of child-bearing age take an iron supplement to protect herself against this condition.

### *Running Performance and the Menstrual Cycle*

Since running has generally beneficial effects on the menstrual period, what about the other side of the cyclic coin? Menstruation causes several physiological changes which can affect performance, including:

- Estrogen-induced water retention can mean premenstrual weight gain of several pounds, which peaks at the beginning of the period and drops steadily through the eighth day.
- Blood values for red blood cell concentration (hematocrit) are lowest at the onset of the period and highest at the time of ovulation.
- There is a distinctly slower reaction time during the premenstrual phase.

* If you are skeptical about this old-fashioned remedy, recent medical research cites aspirin as a safe and potent drug to prevent formation of prostaglandins (a special group of cyclic fatty acids). The prostaglandins are compounds that seem to be ubiquitous in the body and are involved in such unpleasant problems as inflammatory reactions, headache — and muscle and menstrual cramps.

On the basis of these changes, it would seem logical to expect performance to be best during the postmenstrual phase, and at its worst just before and during the menstrual period.

Studies on this subject offer conflicting views. Several support the traditional lower-performance analysis, but in a more recent study nearly half the subjects (46 per cent) reported no significant difference in running ability in any of the phases.*

For the serious athlete, however, *any* variation is important. In the interest of enhancing performance, it's been suggested that oral contraceptives might be effectively used to regulate and even to alter the athlete's cycle, enabling her to compete during the most advantageous phase. Aside from the controversial ethics of this practice, it's also counterproductive. Dr. Shangold points out that the unfavorable conditions that naturally occur in the premenstrual phase (when estrogen and progesterone levels are high) are mimicked and even exaggerated in the pill-user, because her estrogen and progesterone concentrations are even higher during the entire three weeks she is taking the pill. Thus the users of contraceptive pills are at the disadvantage of the premenstrual phase throughout their cycle. Clearly, the "pill" might not be the optimal method of contraception for the serious athlete.

### *The Postmenopausal Woman*

When her periods diminish and then cease, a woman must face two side effects of the menopause: she becomes more susceptible to heart attacks when she loses estrogen's protective effect on the cardiovascular system, and she may develop osteoporosis. Osteoporosis is a condition in which

* See Marge Albohm's article, "Does Menstruation Affect Performance in Sports?" in the March 1976 issue of *The Physician and Sportsmedicine.*

calcium leaches out of the bones, leaving them brittle and vulnerable to breakage.

Dr. Shangold believes that any woman over forty should have a stress test before she embarks on a running program and acknowledges that a woman runs a greater risk of developing stress fractures after menopause. She also points out, however, that there are women of sixty, seventy, and even eighty who run every day with no adverse effects. "On a strictly intuitive level, I would say that a postmenopausal woman who runs would have *fewer* cardiovascular problems and fewer psychological problems too. In this case I believe the benefits of the exercise outweigh the potential hazards."

## Pregnancy

It used to be taken for granted that pregnancy put an instant stop to all strenuous physical activity, and that the pregnant woman would spend nine months in sedentary limbo. This view began to be seriously challenged as the natural childbirth movement taught women that:

- pregnancy and delivery are normal, healthy events, despite the aura of pathology that the hospital setting sometimes creates.
- a high level of fitness provides both physical and emotional support for the birth process.

The modern woman feels free to exercise through most of her pregnancy if she's generally healthy, and if there are *no unusual circumstances*. My second pregnancy fell (resoundingly) into that latter category. Even before I knew *how* unusual my circumstances were, I had to give up hitting tennis balls against the wall. I knew the twinges and pelvic floor pressures I was experiencing were excessive for the fourth month. I lasted a bit longer on the bicycle, limiting my rides to flat ground inside a New York City park. Between my condition and Samantha on the kiddie seat, I was carrying 60 pounds of progeny! It was a tight squeeze behind the handlebars when I finally decided to quit bicycling — and the decision had some positive reinforcement from Jim and my obstetrician.

Admittedly, my case was exceptional. I think a pregnant woman should be guided by her obstetrician's verdict on exercise — if those reasons seem sensible and satisfactory. Presumably she will have placed herself in a physician's care after discussing her attitudes and expectations of the pregnancy and delivery with him/her and will know their views are compatible.

### *The Effects of Running on Pregnancy*

To understand the effects of running on the pregnant body, you have to examine the general effects of pregnancy and realize that running represents an additional workload. As the term "carrying the baby" implies, the principal burdens of pregnancy are the additional weight of the developing infant and the efforts of the body to provide for the infant's nutritional needs. Both of these tax a woman's ability to deliver more blood and oxygen rapidly to her enlarged body. In other words, pregnancy puts additional demands on her cardiovascular-respiratory system. To meet these demands, her cardiac output (amount of blood pumped per minute) goes up by about one third. It does this by increasing the pulse rate (roughly elevated 15 beats per minute) and the stroke volume (the volume of blood ejected with each beat). The total blood volume also begins to rise from the first trimester on. Since the increase in red blood cell mass does *not* keep pace with the increase in plasma volume, the relative concentration of red blood cells and the hemoglobin both drop in what is known as the physiological anemia of pregnancy. (This reduced ability to transport oxygen is offset by a mechanism that allows oxygen to be released more easily from the red blood cells to meet the needs of the tissues.) The overall effect of all these CVR changes enables the pregnant woman to meet the additional demands of her pregnancy.

The CVR responses to pregnancy are similar to those elicited by running — both tax the body to deliver more oxygen to accomplish the additional work. What is important for the pregnant runner to know is that the demands (especially the oxygen demands) of her pregnancy will be supplied first, and that the uterus is virtually assured of good blood supply. Whatever oxygen is *left over* will then be used for the running. For this reason, the uterus has been called a "low resistance shunt." While this safety device is a good thing for the baby in the womb, it also means that the pregnant runner cannot go as fast as she could before, *nor should she even try* because of the additional oxygen demands relating to the pregnancy. Both my pregnancies offered dramatic proof of this "safety valve." Both times I experienced profuse nosebleeds, and by the time I received emergency blood transfusions, my red cell count (hematocrit) was down to half of what it should have been (even allowing for the physiological anemia of pregnancy). When this happened during the first pregnancy, my obstetrician told me not to worry: I might be feeling totally depleted by the "local oxygen shortage," but the baby's needs were being met. He was right — Samantha arrived on time and in glowing good health.

Dr. Shangold feels it's probably all right for the average woman to maintain her pre-pregnancy level of exertion but suggests modifications for women at the low end of the activity scale; sedentary women would benefit from mild, gradual exercise like walking. She adds that serious athletes would be wise to cut back on their training and curtail intensive, anaerobic workouts. Any exercise program during pregnancy should also be adjusted to allow for the gradual weight gain of up to 30 pounds.

### *Running's Effect on Pregnancy and Delivery*

Physical fitness benefits both the mother-to-be and the unborn child. In one Scandinavian study that closely monitored both mothers and babies before and after delivery, the fit mothers showed fewer signs of physiological stress during the course of the labor. One key indication of this was the fact that these women were better able to maintain the normal acid-base (pH) balance of the blood — and their babies shared this advantage. The greater aerobic capacity of the mothers reduced the danger of asphyxiation in the infants during delivery.

Exercise is generally beneficial to expectant women with varicose veins, since the contraction of the leg muscles promotes circulation. The fit mother is also less subject to backache, fatigue, and insomnia — and the woman who runs has less constipation throughout the pregnancy. Insomnia is lessened, too. Exercise alleviates some of the psychological strains of pregnancy, and the tranquil woman sleeps better (in spite of the bulk she's shifting around).

"Labor and delivery are hard work," Dr. Shangold says. "In the same way that a woman who's fit can handle *any* workload better, she can handle labor and delivery in a superior way . . . and with less stress to the baby. A healthy woman with a healthy pregnancy and a healthy placenta who's been used to long distance running, should be able to run right up to the time she delivers. She will have to slow down because the body is doing more work just in terms of the pregnancy . . . and because she's carrying the extra weight. Because of the displacement of the center of gravity . . . and the attendant back strain . . . she may feel uncomfortable running as the pregnancy progresses.

"I think she's best guided by the reactions of her body. A pregnant woman should be *listening* to her body. If she has any medical problems . . . hypertension, bleeding, or anything else . . . she should be *resting,* not running. In any case, a pregnant woman should *not* just go out and run . . . she should ask her obstetrician first. If she develops pain, bleeding, or rupture of the membranes at any time, she should cease training immediately and consult her obstetrician."

*Postpartum Running*

Mary Dono ran until she was five months pregnant and her obstetrician told her she was having twins. Throughout her pregnancy she had lots of energy, no constipation, and only gained 23 pounds (the twins weighed in at 6 pounds, 3 ounces and 6 pounds, 10 ounces). Mary delivered the babies using natural childbirth, and had no medication during an active labor which lasted from 10 A.M. to 7 P.M. The twins were born in May and she was walking-running within two weeks. "I walked five miles at first, then I alternately walked one mile and ran a half mile. I gradually increased those distances, and in six weeks I could run four miles without walking. In September, four months after the birth, I ran a 12.8-mile race."

Extraordinary? Not really, because Mary is one of a growing number of women who know how physical fitness — and running in particular — can ease them through the process of pregnancy and birth. Mary feels her years of running were there with her — helping — in the delivery room. "I felt strong . . . my muscle tone was good . . . and I was completely in charge of the birth. All that is due to the effort and discipline of running. When you run you get into the habit of saying to yourself, 'You can do it.' That habit helps in other life situations too . . . especially in childbirth."

After the birth, Mary had resumed her running prudently.

Alternately walking-and-running is a fine technique for adapting the body to strenuous activity again, and many women have used this method after childbirth — or after an illness or surgery. Let pain be your guide to postpartum running. When the episiotomy has healed you can think about walking-running. Pain is evidence that the healing is not complete, and the running should wait a bit.

*Nursing*

Adequate fluid intake is an important concern for the distance runner, particularly in hot weather. In the nursing mother, fluid intake is vital. Not only must she replace what is lost (through sweat) in the training runs, but she must take in enough additional fluid to make milk. A fully breast-fed baby can easily be consuming a quart of breast milk a day (or the equivalent of two pounds of fluid by weight). So if you are running and nursing, drink, drink, drink!

Denise Conlon nursed her daughter Danielle and also ran every day. She felt good doing both. "People tell you that running is too much of a drain on your energy and that you won't have enough milk," Denise says, "but I think that's an old-wives' tale. I felt fine all along, and I had an abundance of milk." Denise suggests nursing before you run — your breasts will feel more comfortable and you'll know you're not leaving a fussy baby behind with your husband or sitter. "When you're nursing you're home a lot," Denise adds. "It's so easy to just sit there and forget the outside world exists . . . to fall into the baby's sleepy patterns. Running is refreshing. It gets you out of the house for a change of scene, and gives you some time of your own."

If excess weight gain was a problem during your pregnancy, running plus nursing should be a powerful one-two combination to help you recover your figure. This route is far safer than dieting — any concentrated efforts to diet should wait until weaning has well begun. When you are nursing you're responsible for meeting your infant's nutritional needs in a direct and immediate way. The nursing period is not the time to embark on a diet that might shortchange either you or your baby.

The calorie arithmetic of running plus nursing is good news for everyone. It takes roughly a thousand calories to make a quart of milk. If you add to this the nearly one hundred calories consumed by each mile of running, you can see that running-nursing puts you on an effective "diet" without any further calorie restrictions.

When you begin to run again, don't overdo. A new mother may be as anxious to recover her pre-pregnancy running form as her pre-pregnancy shape. Since she may have dropped 25 pounds with the birth, she's likely to feel she has wings on her heels. Psychologically, she may be yearning to claim her body as her own again. Making your body comply with exacting demands is a clear-cut way of reclaiming it.

There's no harm if eagerness to run again is tempered by a sensible approach. Limit the frequency of hard anaerobic workouts. Race if you like, but don't make an all-out racing effort every weekend. You might temporarily succeed in handling the stress, but fatigue would catch up. One of the most important ingredients in any increased running program is lots of rest — which new mothers rarely enjoy — and chronic exhaustion can be sharply disruptive to breastfeeding. (After the birth of the quads, my pediatrician insisted that I sleep and let the nurse bottle-feed the babies at 2 A.M. — on the grounds that I needed to rest *sometime* in order to make more milk.)

Few other things in life are as special as the delicately synchronized relationship of the new mother and her nursing baby. Don't jeopardize this experience by trying to do too much too soon. You've waited nine months to get where you are, so enjoy it.

EIGHT

# RUNNING AND YOUR MIND

## *Emotional Benefits, the Runner's "High," and Danger Signals*

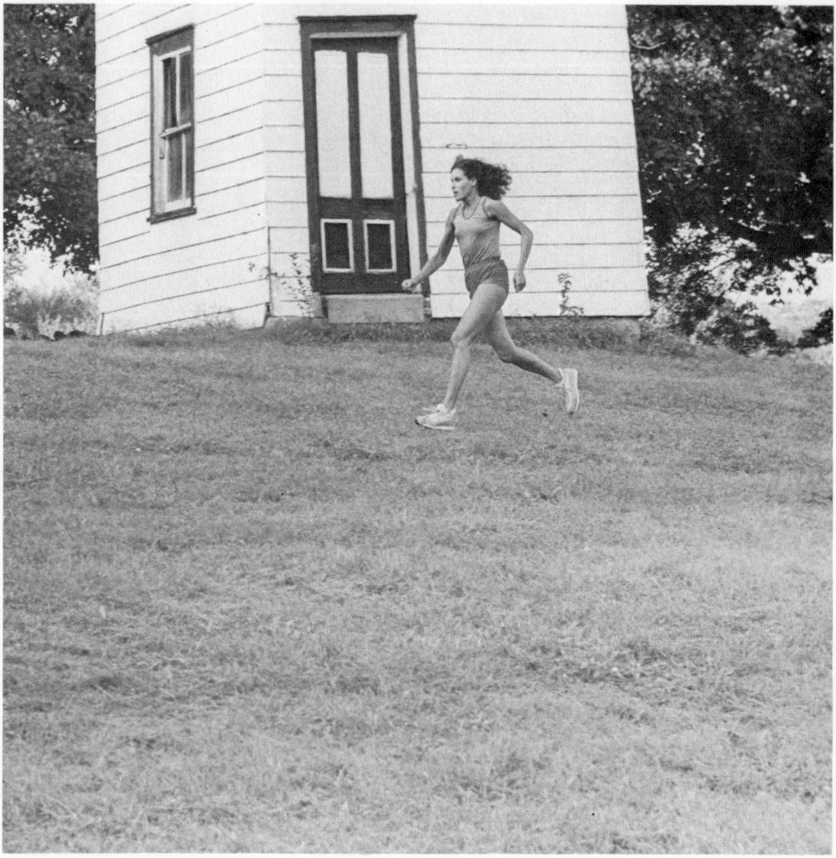

A mellow afternoon — a tranquil run. *Melchior DiGiacomo*

Sometimes when I am running I wonder which is benefiting most — my body or my mind. I may have started the run mulling over some problem with the kids, or gnawing on one of those logistical conundrums that plague the car-pooling suburban mother. As time and distance pass, however, and I tune into the rhythmic sensations of the run, I find I can't hold on to even the most persistent worries. They simply fade away. What takes their place is the free association of the road — floating thoughts that drift in and out, recollections, memories of things that happened years ago. When I get home my problem may still be with me — I know it hasn't been resolved — but this "emptying out" of my head has dissipated all the tension.

The thoughts that course through the mind during a run can range from the purely prosaic to the ethereal. They may deal with practical subjects like planning the day, may help with problem-solving, or may be registering a sensory appreciation of the runner's surroundings that translates into joy.

Every woman I've interviewed has stated that the emotional boost she derived from her runs equaled — or surpassed — the physical gains. Jim Fixx says that "The qualities and capacities that are important in running — such factors as will power, the ability to apply effort during extreme fatigue, and the acceptance of pain — have a radiating power that subtly influences one's life." Running's psychological dividends varied with the individual, but there were basic touchstones, among them:

- *Increased Self-confidence and Self-esteem.* As the runner begins to have evidence of the physical benefits of the running, she also begins to have more positive feelings about herself. Her self-esteem grows, and so does her poise in social situations.
- *Peace of Mind.* The solitude of running gives the mind "breathing space," a time when a woman may either grapple with the issues in her life, or simply let her mind rest. In the sense that it allows the time for both confrontation *and* coasting, running promotes inner peace.
- *Control of Her Life.* Because she's tested it with speed and distance, a runner feels in control of her body and, by extension, in control of her life. All the tenacity and self-discipline she summoned in order to do well at running serves her splendidly in everyday situations, and the regularity of her runs invests her life with a sense of stability and a predictable rhythm.
- *Relief of Tension.* Running functions admirably as an antidote to tension and anxiety. It's well-known that the sport brings psychological relief to many — young mothers besieged with family responsibilities, career women with heavy family-job schedules, and the woman who finds herself alone. In this latter category are many who feel "displaced" because of divorce, widowhood, or the fact that their children are grown. Running can do a remarkable job of bolstering the spirits of the displaced woman — making her physically healthier, strengthening her emotional outlook, and building her self-esteem.

- *Practical Advantages.* Many women use their morning run to simply perk up after a full night's sleep — to make marketing lists in their heads, mentally sift through their wardrobes, and plan their time. They use their runs to "order" their days.
- *Playfulness.* Running allows a woman to be in touch with the inner child — to indulge in fantasies, shed inhibitions, and savor the freedom of her workouts.
- *The Spiritual Aspect.* Each woman I interviewed tried to frame the meaning of her running in terms of her own existence — some would speak of a heightened awareness, some would describe feelings of closeness to God and nature as they ran along. Most were affected in distinctly spiritual ways, but it was a spirituality largely derived from the (often poignant) realization of their own potential. None spoke of running as a surrogate religion. The spiritual insight generated by running does not have to fit into a religious framework — but it is certainly not incompatible with formal religion, and can enhance a religious perspective.

## The Runner's High

The most nebulous, but often-mentioned, facet of running is the "runner's high" — a kind of euphoria that can range from simple feelings of well-being to an altered state of consciousness (with a wide spectrum of emotions in between). Those who do report this altered (almost mystical) perspective say it seems to happen 30 or 40 minutes into the run.

Psychiatrist-runner Thaddeus Kostrubala believes that the repetitive action of slow distance running eventually fatigues the area of the brain (the motor cortex) that normally controls voluntary motor activity. He thinks that when this area tires, the activity is referred to lower brain centers, which sustain it. As long as the running is directed by the voluntary motor cortex, it feels like hard work, but once control is shifted to the lower brain centers — within 30 or 40 minutes — the sense of physical effort is gone. It's like going on an automatic pilot — the runner feels as if she were in a continuum and could go on forever. Regular running may permit the consciousness to glimpse the functions of the right side of the brain, which Dr. Kostrubala says are "intuitive, aesthetic, creative, nonlogical, and nonsequential and which seem to escape the temporal order of things."

One of the most interesting attempts to provide a biomechanical explanation for the psychological effects of running is the theory advanced by Dr. Arnold Mandell, professor of psychiatry at the University of California Medical School at San Diego. Dr. Mandell believes that runners not only feel a "second wind" about thirty minutes into the run, but also experience a *second* "second wind" sometime after the first hour of the run. Dr. Mandell calls the first episode at the 30-minute mark largely physical, "legs and arms become light and rhythmic . . . the fatigue goes away, and feelings of power begin." He describes the second energy shift as close to mystical: "Colors are bright and beautiful, water sparkles, clouds breathe, and my body, swimming, detaches from the earth. A loving contentment invades the basement of my mind, and thoughts bubble up in trails. In the long distance runner, the *second* second wind is beyond pain, hunger, thirst, anger, or depression: transcendent."

Dr. Mandell connects these phenomena with neurochemical events in the brain. Like Dr. Kostrubala, he suggests an alteration in the relationship between the right and left hemispheres of the brain. He thinks it is "likely that each temporal lobe represents a different world view" (verbal-analytic on the left and visual-intuitive on the right).

In relation to the first "second wind," Dr. Mandell suggests that running influences the expression of consciousness on each side of the brain. He speculates that this mechanism involves seratonin* metabolism and its level of distribution to each hemisphere of the brain, resulting in what he terms "release of right-lobe optimism." (In Dr. Mandell's case the "optimism" involved thoughts of a doubled research grant request, or visions of running 25 miles.)

Dr. Mandell theorizes that, during the second "second wind," the seratonin production shuts off completely because of the sensitive feedback system that causes seratonin to inhibit its own manufacture. The modifying effect of seratonin is then arrested, allowing both brain hemispheres free expression. Dr. Mandell believes the result is a surge of psychic activity that involves "an awareness of both sides at once," providing "high energy bliss."

## The Runner as "Addict"

There are runners who are so devoted to the sport that they compare their workouts to an addict's "fix." They're being facetious, of course, but many experts believe that running can indeed be physically addictive.

Dr. Kostrubala observes that runners who cannot be active for some reason often feel heavy pressure to go out and run nevertheless, and may "start developing an intense depression." He thinks that a runner may become addicted if he/she runs for one hour three times a week at 75 to 80 per cent of his/her maximum cardiac output. Dr. Mandell echoes the belief that "if you run 6 miles a day for two months, you are addicted forever."

* Seratonin is a chemical substance that performs many functions in the body. In the brain, where it is present in large concentrations, it is involved in many neurochemical processes and seems to play a role in transmitting or modifying nervous signals.

Dr. William Morgan, professor of physical education and director of the Sport Psychology Laboratory at the University of Wisconsin, says running "should be viewed as a wonder drug. It has profound potential in preventing mental and physical disease and in rehabilitation after various illnesses have occurred. However, just like other wonder drugs, running has the potential for abuse, and the runner who appears in the physician's office on crutches or in a wheelchair as a result of the crippling effects of excessive running can be compared to the hard-core drug addict who overdoses. Running is a form of negative addiction in the case of the hard-core exercise addict."

Many medical-running authorities believe that running as an addiction has a biochemical base and is triggered by endorphins — substances that mimic the effects of morphine. Endorphins are manufactured in various parts of the brain, but interestingly only those areas called the "old brain" that man shares with the lower animals (areas affecting mood, for instance). Laboratory research indicates that endorphins work effectively as pain killers, but whether they are the reason for the runner's euphoria has not yet been proven.

Sharp insights into running addiction are offered by Dr. Michael Sacks: "I think running when you are hurt is a major signal . . . it indicates that you are unable to listen to the messages from your body. If life itself seems to become an intrusion on your running, so that you skip important meetings or break social engagements in order to run . . . things may be going wrong. A chronic state of exhaustion would be another clue, and so would lack of flexibility . . . the inability to take off a day or two."

The principles of moderation should be applied to running as to anything else. Running in severe pain or exhaustion goes beyond diligent and disciplined effort — beyond the admirable determination that enables runners to race. Dr. Sacks says, "There's a clear difference between the point where exercise energizes and exercise exhausts." This is something each runner must determine for herself by a candid appraisal of her physical condition and an honest evaluation of her training habits.

## Running — or Running Away?

I've often heard the comment that when I am running, I'm running away from home (and the strain of caring for a big, busy family). My answer is that this is partly true — but then I always run home again! For most women, running is a combination of physical and emotional ingredients. They are happy about the sheer pleasure of their runs, happy that they're improving their health, and — yes — happy to temporarily escape from the duties and problems of wifehood and motherhood. Like me, most feel fortified by the workout, and are glad to be running through their front doors again. If they're *not* pleased to be home, they may be in trouble.

Running is usually a solitary act, and it takes time. The amount of time one spends on running is elective — the beginner may run only 20 or 25 minutes three times a week, a more seasoned runner may need an hour a day, and the woman preparing for a marathon may be training many hours each week. This time has to be subtracted from that spent in other pursuits — from school, from a job, from the family.

The woman who doubles or triples her usual daily run and chooses to work out in "prime family time" (weekends, for instance) may be using her running as a "distancing" device. She could be ignoring marital or other family conflicts by putting miles between herself and the involved family member. She may be using running as an antidote for depression or a free-floating anxiety. Or she may be using time for running instead of using it to deal with family relationships in a meaningful way — thus abdicating her responsibilities.

Obviously none of this applies to the woman who runs out of an occasional family conflict for a healthy period of "cooling off" — who uses running as a constructive tension reliever — or who eases into the emotional flow of her family right after her run. The signs of "distancing" are more pronounced and have an unconscious common aim of pushing aside serious underlying problems. Instead of ignoring physical pain, the runner is ignoring emotional stress. Remedies for this situation might vary from a frank discussion with the rest of the family to professional therapy, but the woman concerned must *recognize* the pattern first.

Some of the women interviewed for this book ran as little as 10 miles a week, some ran more than 70. Most got all they wanted from the sport without compromising family relationships or other activities. There were plenty of frustrations about botched days and juggled schedules, but these women generally managed to keep their running — and their lives — in good perspective.

NINE

# FUELS, FOLLIES, AND HEALTH

## *Diet, Weight Control, Smoking, and Sex*

A runner quickly realizes that everything she puts into her mouth becomes body fuel — and she usually begins to scrutinize her intake. As running makes you aware of your muscles, your heartbeat, your breathing, it also makes you aware of your digestive tract. After all, if health is the object, what's the point of tuning up with high-quality exercise, then undoing the effort by eating junk food?

A good runner's diet is one that's nutritionally sound, and it may have some striking characteristics. Speak to a hundred runners, for instance, and a *very* large percentage will tell you they eat little meat — or none. Though there may be more complicated physiological reasons for the runner's general aversion to meat, the ones that come to mind are simple: meat feels heavy in the stomach and is harder to digest. Runners find they feel better (specifically *lighter*) without it — get out of the habit of eating it — and then find it's not missed.

Freya Block and Phyllis Cantor are typical of this pattern — the more they ran, the less they cared to eat meat. "I just have no desire for it now," Freya says. She eats poultry and fish instead, more dairy products, and an abundance of fresh fruits and vegetables. Phyllis believes she may eat more now than in her pre-running days. "When I first started running, I became much more careful about my diet. I'm sure I eat more food now, but it's better food." Phyllis has a teen-age daughter who's a vegetarian. "We tend to follow her preferences . . . no meat or chicken, but plenty of fish, dairy products, grains, vegetables and fruit."

I stopped eating meat on a regular basis ten years ago, at the time of my first pregnancy. It seemed difficult to digest, and I felt heavy enough with the baby. A month after Samantha was born, I had an outdoor barbecue for the family. When that classic American culinary object — the giant steak — was plopped down in front of me, I realized I couldn't eat it, that I had no appetite for red meat at all. The feeling persisted. With inflation increasing, a steak may soon be the classic American artifact, but that doesn't bother me or my family. There are many less expensive and more satisfactory ways of obtaining protein.

Though there are the usual candy-bar addicts and beer guzzlers among runners, most of us tend to eat well. "Eating well" means partaking of the nutritionally approved food groups — fruits, vegetables, whole grains, eggs,* milk products, legumes, seeds and nuts, fish, poultry, and (for some) meat — while avoiding useless (and possibly harmful) foods like greasy french-fries, sugar-laden colas, and fast-food hamburgers.

Many runners and other athletes are "ovo-lacto" vegetarians, meaning that they eat eggs and dairy products as well as the basic vegetarian foods — grains, nuts and seeds, vegetables, fruits, and legumes (beans and lentils). They avoid protein deficiencies by combining foods to achieve

* Eggs are high in cholesterol, and high blood cholesterol may increase the chance of heart attack and stroke (men and postmenopausal women are particularly vulnerable to both). On the other hand, eggs are a complete protein. I use them freely when cooking (from cakes to casseroles) for the children, but try to keep a strict quota on Jim's consumption.

the essential amino acid couples: milk products with grains (whole-grain cereal and milk), grains with legumes (rice and beans), and legumes with nuts and seeds (beans with sesame seeds).*

In making meals for myself and my family, I don't pay homage to a single diet philosophy. I tend to plan intuitively, using common sense and a basic knowledge of nutrition as my guides. We eat chicken and fresh fish (although the kids still prefer canned tuna), vegetables, fruits, eggs, and dairy products — skim milk, yogurt, and cottage cheese (and less often cheese with higher fat content). I use grains, nuts, and seeds liberally with other foods — adding cooked and seasoned wheat flakes to any pasta or noodle dish, topping casseroles with a crumb-like mixture of wheat germ (or bran), finely chopped nuts, sunflower seeds, and grated cheese — or I might toss this combination on top of our salads. I've gradually developed a recipe for "meat loaf" that has become virtually meatless — thanks to increasing proportions of soaked and seasoned cracked soy granules, wheat germ (or bran), a variety of nuts and seeds (chopped peanuts and sunflower seeds), chopped celery, scallions, beaten eggs (to bind everything together), and a *small* amount of lean, ground beef.

Most of my kitchen experimenting is of the "applied research" variety — adapting favorite recipes to simplify their preparation and also to find healthier substitutes for certain ingredients. Yogurt successfully replaces sour cream, for instance, even in my favorite banana cake recipe — and thoroughly blended cottage cheese pinch-hits for cream cheese in dips, spreads, and cheesecake. I add wheat germ and non-fat dry milk powder almost anywhere I can, and

* How the protein sources complement each other is fully explained in Frances Moore Lappé's vegetarian bible, *Diet for a Small Planet* (New York: Ballantine Books, 1971).

I like to make my own granola (accenting our favorite ingredients such as mixed dried fruits, pineapple, and coconut shreds, nuts, plus sesame seeds for flavor and crunch). I've found bread baking isn't all that complex or time consuming (it only requires my attention periodically), and I've finally gotten it down to an inexact science. I enjoy baking bread, but I don't do it consistently — to keep my family supplied, I'd have to turn the kitchen into a nonstop bakery. Our breads — home-baked or store-bought — are the whole grain variety.

Women who run are usually keenly aware of the interplay between good nutrition and good health. They improve their own diets, then examine their family's diet as well. Cans of tinted "juices," potato chips, candy, and instant (chemical) "soups" disappear from their larders and are replaced by foods with better nutritional value — and better dollar value as well. Good nutrition is a health dividend for the family with a running mother.

## Vitamins for Running

There are runners who try every dietary supplement from traditional ones like cod-liver oil and brewer's yeast to the more exotic bee-pollen and ginseng. But barring the unlikely possibility of a serious diet deficiency, runners have pretty much the same nutritional needs as the rest of the (nonrunning) population. It's not true, for instance, that a runner needs more protein than a sedentary person — unless the runner happens to be pregnant or nursing. (Indeed, consumption of too much protein can be dangerous — taxing the kidneys and excretory system, which have to cope with the excess.) All other runners can be guided by the RDA (recommended daily allowance) standards which set the daily protein requirement at 46 grams for a woman and 56 grams for a man.

There *are* several nutrients which runners seem to require in larger amounts than nonrunners — Vitamin C, for one. Vitamin C is important in the manufacture of collagen, a protein found in loose connective tissue in the form of long, wavy, nonelastic strands. Since connective tissue in various areas of the body can be subject to injury, some running authorities recommend taking one gram (1000mg.) of Vitamin C for each hour of running. Dr. Kostrubala believes that Vitamin C helps ward off fatigue and illness as well.

Vitamin E is also recommended for runners, primarily because of its antioxidant properties, but also because naturally occurring Vitamin E is processed out of most foods. Refined flours are degerminated to enhance their "shelf-life," and although subsequent enriching adds some of the B vitamins and iron, it does not replace lost Vitamin E or trace minerals.

Recent Vitamin A research should be of special interest to urban runners who listen for daily air quality announcements or suburban runners who can't avoid rush hour traffic. "Bad air" taxes the breathing apparatus when carbon monoxide, ozone, and other pollutants clog the filtering system that lines the respiratory passages. This natural purifying system consists of fine, hairlike projections (cilia) that beat rhythmically to move the mucus and trapped foreign particles in the direction of the nose and mouth. When too many pollutants get caught in the mucus, it hampers the action of the cilia. The good news is that there's now experimental evidence showing that Vitamin A plays a significant role in keeping these particular tissues in a healthy state. Including Vitamin A in the diet can be done without resorting to supplements — a single cupful of cooked carrots provides 16,000 I.U. (international units) or 80 per cent of the RDA.

It also appears that exercise itself helps your body fight pollution. A study conducted on runners who trained during peak traffic hours showed that although they inhaled about 40 per cent more pollutants, the runners also *excreted* more. As a result, they finished the study with some 20 per cent less lead in their systems than a sedentary control group. Just as endurance training increases the body's capacity to process oxygen and rid itself of the (metabolic) waste products of exercise, so it also improves the body's ability to cast off foreign (inhaled) pollutants. Moral: air pollution is *not* a good reason for avoiding exercise.

## The Weigh-in — Running and Weight Control

Serious dieters used to avoid exercise for two reasons now known to be myths. They assumed that exercise burns up too few calories to make the effort worthwhile, and they were afraid that the exercise would so increase their appetite that they would finally gain weight rather than lose it.

Both myths are roundly scotched by Dr. Jean Mayer, former professor of nutrition at Harvard University and now president of Tufts University. Dr. Mayer maintains that exercise *does* play an important part in weight control. "Persons of the same height and weight maintain that weight on radically different levels of calorie intake when their regimens of physical activity are different. Prolonged exercise does make you hungrier, but not so hungry that you eat more calories than you've used up."

*Any* combination of dieting and exercise that adds up to a calorie deficit will result in lost pounds. The arithmetic of weight loss takes no notice of whether the calorie reduction is accomplished by eating less or exercising more — or both.

Women who want to incorporate exercise into a weight-loss program should have some information on the calorie cost of running. The usual figure of 100 calories consumed for every mile you run is accurate only if you weigh 150 pounds and run somewhat slower than an 8-minute per mile pace. The rate at which calories are used varies only slightly with the speed of the runner. If you are running 6-minute miles, you'll cover 5 miles in half an hour. If you're running 12-minute miles, you'll cover 2½ miles in that same half hour. Obviously you're burning twice as many calories at a 6-minute pace. A more typical range would be between an 8-minute mile and a 10-minute mile. During a 40-minute run, the 8-minute miler will cover 5 miles, while the 10-minute miler covers 4. If you weigh under 130 pounds, the net difference is less than 90 calories consumed.

The more important variable in the 100 calories per mile approximation is not speed, but body weight. It requires more energy (calories) to move a greater mass. The overweight person is usually carrying most of her extra weight in the form of fat which — unlike muscle — is nonworking weight. Exercise is even harder at this point because the muscles are heavily taxed to carry "the dead weight" of the fat. Therefore the difference in calorie consumption between a 120-pound and a 180-pound runner (both moving at an 8-minute pace) is sizable. Because of this factor, weight loss is more dramatic in the early stages of the diet-exercise program than it is later on, when the ideal weight is approached.

As the calorie-counting runner continues to lose weight (and the level of diet and exercise remain the same), the rate of weight loss will slow down and gradually taper off. Each decrease in weight means it will take fewer calories to maintain the reduced body weight and also require a greater calorie deficit to obtain the same weight loss. For every 10 pounds of weight lost, the dieter will burn 6 to 8 fewer calories when running a mile, and she will require roughly 150 fewer calories on a daily basis to maintain her new body weight. Clearly, her weight will stabilize at some point unless she runs longer, or eats less, or both.

The arithmetic of calorie-counting does not tell the whole story of weight control. We've been dealing with the simple law of conservation of matter (weight) and energy (calories). What we haven't considered are the individual variations in body composition (relative proportions of lean weight and fat) and in body chemistry (metabolism) that account for the differences in the ways our bodies process calories.

*Body Composition*

An enigma that drives the overweight to the brink of despair is this: two people weigh the same and consume the same number of daily calories — yet one gains weight and the other does not. Exercise physiologists are beginning to understand the causes of dilemmas like these, and their explanations should help us revise some of our thinking about what it means to be "overweight" or "underweight." The medical researchers in exercise physiology think of the body as being divided into two parts: fat and lean body mass (LBM),* which consists of lean muscle, bones, and tissue.

Instead of thinking in terms of an ideal body weight based on the usual factors (height, build, age, etc.), it's now believed to be more accurate to project an ideal body weight by calculating a person's LBM and adding the appropriate fat allowances — 15 per cent for a man, 22 per cent for a woman.† This distinction is important because it means we should now think in terms of "overfat" or "un-

* The fact that fat is less dense and floats, while LBM sinks, is the basis for the underwater immersion test to determine percentage of body fat. The thinner you are, the denser you are, and the heavier you will tip the underwater scales — that is, the closer your underwater weight approaches your regular weight, the smaller the fat percentage will be.

† According to Covert Bailey in *Fit or Fat?* (Boston: Houghton Mifflin Company, 1978), these percentages represent the upper limits of the normal (healthy) range, though both figures are well below average for the American male and female.

derfat," and keep in mind that it's possible to be underweight according to the traditional charts and still be overfat — and also to be overweight and underfat. (Professional athletes, like football players, tend to be victims of the old approach. Uninformed coaches chide them when they tip the scales, but often the average player's total weight is high in muscle, *low* in fat.) This method of calculation also means that ideal weight is not a number fixed for all time — it varies as a function of an individual's LBM.

The problem is that many doctors, nutritionists, and dieters are still transfixed by the notion of ideal body weight, and are chained to what physician-runner-author Joan Ullyot calls, "the tyranny of the bathroom scales." Understanding the body's division into fat and LBM helps us clarify the conditioning effects caused by running, and understand how these affect weight control.

It's important to keep in mind that your lean body mass is the proper basis for determining your daily calorie allowance. This makes good sense since the LBM is the part of your body that does all the work and uses the calories, while the body's fat gets a free ride — it doesn't need calories because it does no work. This fact solves the two-people–same-calorie-intake puzzle: the calorie utilization difference is understandable if there's a difference in how their weight is distributed between LBM and fat. The person with a higher percentage of fat (smaller LBM and lower calorie requirement) would show a weight gain, while the leaner person would hold steady on the same diet. The leaner person would also inevitably be the *exercising* body — the working muscles strengthen and increase in mass (LBM)* while body fat is substantially reduced (usually with a net loss in weight).

* This does not mean increase in muscle bulk. With training, the intramuscular fat that is marbled throughout the lean muscle tissue is burned off and replaced with additional lean muscle tissue.

Recent research points to the superiority of a weight loss program stressing *both* diet and exercise. The combined program is better not because those tested had a higher weight loss,* but because the subjects who exercised while they dieted lost more *fat* and gained more *lean tissue*.

*Muscle Metabolism*

Apart from body composition, exercise training also affects body metabolism — especially the energy-producing chemical processes that go on inside the muscle cells. Training coordinates changes on several levels so that the body can process more oxygen and increase its capacity to work even harder.

It now appears that the *individual muscle cell* also increases its aerobic capacity as part of the stepped-up metabolism. Crucial changes occur in its internal chemical processes that concern dieters as well as runners interested in racing performance. Prompted by exercise, the muscle cell switches over to synthesizing the enzymes that will enable it to burn fats more readily (see Fat Utilization in the Appendix). For the dieter this means that the calories taken in are less likely to be turned into fat deposits, and this is the basis for Covert Bailey's belief that "the ultimate cure for obesity is exercise. Exercise increases muscle, tones it, alters its chemistry, and increases the metabolic rate."

The result? You burn more calories even while you sleep. What could be a better diet formula than that?

## The Beauty Dividends

A wish for a better figure is what usually inspires a woman to start running. Once she gets into the sport she quickly

* As a matter of fact, they *did* have higher weight loss, but not one that was statistically significant.

perceives all the fitness benefits, but the old "pounds and inches" are the popular motivators. Once the gritty initial period has passed and she's running with ease and enjoyment, the runner becomes aware that her body is changing its shape. Slowly the fat pads disappear, the muscles firm, the stomach flattens, and she feels lithe again. It's an exhilarating transformation that's recalled with a kind of wonderment by the participants.

Donna Welsh and Lois King are Westchester County, New York, housewives and friends who've been running for several years. Both were concerned about their figures when they began. "I had a good look at myself in the mirror one day, and I felt unhappy," Donna says. "My husband ran for two years before I started . . . his body was lean and mine was getting chubby . . . so I started running myself. I'm not athletic. If I can do it, anyone can. Running has been great for me . . . my whole body shape has changed. When you've had a few children and have mostly been sitting around, you get hippy. Now I'm streamlined. I recently ran into an old college friend who's become quite pudgy, and she couldn't get over the way I looked."

Lois is a slender fashion model who says, "I'd been playing tennis for a number of years, and I enjoyed the exercise, but I gradually became aware that staying tall and *thin* would require more work than tennis provided. I started running with a friend who taught aerobic dancing, and she explained aerobic activity to me. My first time out I ran about 30 feet and said, 'This is absurd. How can I run a mile?' But I persisted through the first six months — dying, hating it, but sticking with it too. Now I love running. I've lost both weight and inches, and people began saying how good I looked. When I run in the morning, I have plenty of energy for both work and tennis later on."

Katie Baxter says she totally reshaped herself through

running. "One summer, when I had more time, I increased my mileage. I didn't notice much difference at first, but after a few months the changes were incredible. I was losing inches and feeling wonderful at the same time. I had made my body into a new machine."

Phyllis Cantor had a similar experience. "After a period of time I noticed a change in the way I looked. I began getting support and reinforcement from family and friends. Word would come back to me that people thought I looked much better and my children said so too. I take the same dress size . . . 12 or 14 . . . but I have a greater choice in that range. My weight seems rearranged."

I'm also happy about what running has done for my figure, even though I'm one of those rare people it's helped by providing a slight weight gain. The year or so after the children were born I was probably too thin. I ate as much as I wanted, but there was so little sleep and so much sheer activity that the calories were being burned off as fast as the food was eaten. I weigh 108 pounds now, which is just about right, and I'm pleased that my body has some lean muscle definition.

One other beauty benefit most runners notice is an improvement in their skin, which seems generally clearer and brighter. Mary Vitiello is a Westchester, New York, runner, a busy model, and the mother of two school-age boys. Mary, who has a beautiful complexion, says, "Makeup could never duplicate the glow that running gives the skin." The "glow" is achieved with the help of the healthy sweat worked up in the course of a vigorous workout. The sweat opens the pores, cleansing them. At the same time, blood is rushed to the surface (to be "air-cooled"), and the skin is stimulated by the increased circulation. Complexions seem to perk up with a running regimen.

## Smoking

Running and smoking don't mix. A smoker who becomes a runner is promptly made aware of their incompatibility: while the act of running is demanding more oxygen, smoking is undermining the body's ability to deliver the oxygen required. Many of the women runners I interviewed are now ex-smokers. They say usually there's no contest — that it's only a matter of weeks or months before the smoking stops. One friend who quit smoking on the eve of his first Boston Marathon subsequently completed the grueling Western States 100-mile run in under 24 hours, without benefit (?) of cigarettes.

## Coffee

There are some runners who shun coffee because it causes them to suffer a battery of discomforts — insomnia, rapid heartbeat, and indigestion — and some who dote on it for its stimulating effects. The ranks of coffee drinkers have received some positive reinforcement from Dr. David Costill, director of the Human Performance Laboratory at Ball State University, Muncie, Indiana. Dr. Costill observed an almost 30 per cent increase in the length of time test subjects could exercise before exhaustion set in when two cups of coffee were taken first.

In a subsequent study where the subjects did not know that they were drinking coffee, the amount of work performed in 2 hours' time increased by about 7 per cent; at the same time, the subjects' sense of effort was diminished. Coffee apparently made more work seem like less. The explanation for this is complex, but it involves caffeine's effect on the relative proportions of glycogen and fat that fuel the exercise. Costill found that caffeine ingestion increased the percentage of energy that derived from the fat from 22 per cent to 40 per cent.*

This increased utilization of fat is particularly significant in long-distance races, because it has the effect of sparing muscle glycogen. As a result, a pre-race cup of coffee (brewed double-strength and taken black a full hour before the run) has been recommended especially to marathon runners as a possible defense against exhaustion in the last stages of the race. For those who don't care to take coffee, Costill suggests a highly caffeinated tea, brewed strong, or caffeine tablets.

The runner unaccustomed to coffee should beware of possible adverse effects. Caffeine can cause diarrhea, and it also acts as a diuretic. This may mean anything from a minor inconvenience of extra stops during a marathon to the serious hazard of dehydration from excess fluid loss in hot-weather racing. Since some smaller individuals (particularly women weighing 100–110 pounds) are easily overdosed by caffeine, Dr. Costill suggests the pre-race intake be limited to no more than 5 mg. of caffeine per kilogram of body weight (roughly two cups of coffee), and suggests the caffeine intake should be tested on training runs several times before the race.

## Sugar

An unfortunate spin-off of the carbohydrate-loading craze is the tendency (especially in first-time marathoners) to

* Caffeine stimulates the sympathetic nervous system, causing fat cells to release more free fatty acids into the blood. However, medical authorities now caution that continuously high levels of free fatty acids may contribute to the development of atherosclerosis, diabetes, and heart disease.

continue the loading phase right up until the start of the race, nibbling on sweets even at the starting line in the mistaken notion that more sugar then means more energy in reserve for the final push. In actual fact, the opposite is true.

Dr. Costill found that runners who drank a sugared drink 30–45 minutes before exercising had greater difficulty running and tired more rapidly. He concluded that eating any sugary food within an hour before the race would only hurt performance — and this warning included the "athletic drinks" because of their sugar content.

The reason for this involves the body's usual mechanism for maintaining blood sugar (glucose) levels within normal range: when sugars are eaten, there is an almost immediate rise in blood glucose. This stimulates the pancreas to release insulin, which is the hormone responsible for the removal of glucose from the bloodstream and for reducing the amount of glucose that is usually available from the glycogen stores in the liver (see Hormonal Changes in Exercise in the Appendix). A runner who approaches the starting line in that condition (with elevated blood insulin) is at a relative disadvantage. If the racer starts to exercise vigorously, the insulin and the muscular activity may combine to remove glucose from the blood at an alarming rate in the first 10 minutes of the running. This process makes the first mile as difficult as the twentieth in a marathon race.

The anti-sugar ban is lifted as soon as the race starts. Once exercise begins, it inhibits the release of insulin, so weak glucose drinks are useful from that point on. Ultramarathoners find it particularly helpful to boost their energy by consuming sugar during a race.

## Running and Sex

Whenever running is mentioned in the same breath as sex, it usually triggers the flippant remark that the runner's greater aerobic capacity provides a greater erotic capacity too. It's too facile to say flatly that running improves sexual performance. The most important sex organ is believed to be the brain, and much of running's influence on sex arrives by that more subtle route.

There's no denying the sensual element in the rhythmic sensations of the body in motion — runners who tune into these signals may experience a new dimension of awareness. Even more dramatic for most women is the sexuality implicit in the mastery of their bodies.

Running allows a woman to claim her body as her own — by working it strenuously she appropriates it. Her body is no longer passive or quiescent as it was before but is more responsive to her wishes and more expressive of her inner self. She's infused with a new sense of unity and wholeness, and this feeling enhances every aspect of her life — including sex.

TEN

# RUNNING AND THE FAMILY

## *Family Fitness, Children's Races, and "Crewing"*

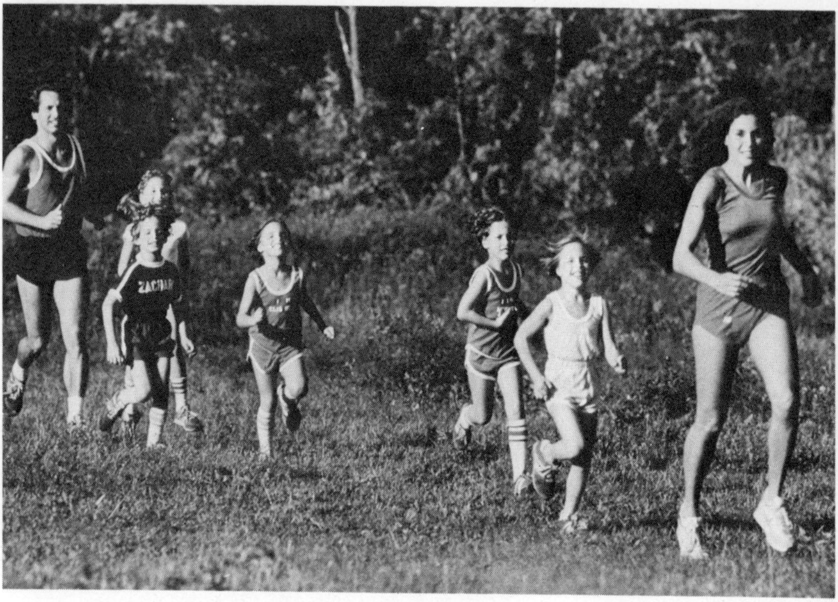

The tribe on the run. *Melchior DiGiacomo*

No woman runs in a vacuum. When she slips into her running shoes and steps out the door, she takes her family with her. They may not be there physically, but they're the beneficiaries of every stride she takes. All the considerable physical and emotional advantages she's gaining are passed along to them.

A mother who runs is sharper about every particular of her family's well-being. She doesn't buy empty, processed foods because she understands the role of nutrition in the maintenance of a physically active body. She has no patience with television hypnosis — her children are not slumped in the darkness, but out in the sunshine *moving*. And she spurs the rest of the family to try their athletic wings.

What happens to a sedentary family when the mother starts to run can be wonderful to see. The father may not care to run himself but will pick up his own level of activity — walking to the train if he's a commuter, or biking or walking to work. Pride is the motivating force that gets him going (can he sit and do *nothing* while his wife is outside running?), and pleasure keeps him at it. Even a modest increase in his level of activity will help a sedentary man tone up his muscles and feel immeasurably better about himself.

The boys and girls begin to stir — joining teams at school, swimming at the Y, trying dance classes and gymnastics. Children who don't think of themselves as "athletic" when they're small, often maintain a poor self-image through all their growing years and into adolescence and adulthood. They may be timid about starting athletic activities, but a running mother helps by her example and her encouragement. (I don't believe in casting children into bitterly competitive athletic situations, and this is particularly true of late starters. It's far better to let them choose their own activity and level of effort.)

The physically active mother can ease her whole family into a more vigorous lifestyle, but she shouldn't try to do so by preaching. Just setting a healthy example is eventually bound to make a dent in the attitudes of her husband and children. When they plainly see how positively exercise works for her, they'll begin to think in terms of shaking a leg and doing something for themselves.

If just *some* family members are reluctant, the canny mother will divide and conquer. Deal with the children first, since they're usually a captive audience. If you are in a suburban or rural situation and must use the car, routinely park it several blocks away from your destination: the inconvenience is overshadowed by the good effects of walking. Get the children out of the habit of thinking that the car is required for every errand. The point is to gently push them to move whenever you get the chance. Don't make a big chore of it, but create an environment that is conducive to walking, to moving, to running around. If your husband is cooperative, but the children are still sluggish, make a point of letting them see Mother and Dad running — or biking — or swimming together. Before long they'll want to participate.

Even bad weather can work to good advantage in keeping everyone in motion. On rainy days, when the children say they are "bored," remember you have a source of cheap labor under your roof. Hand them a broom, a dustcloth, or a bucket. And keep the television set turned *off*. In our house the children must ask permission to turn it on, and *we* pick the shows. I try not to let television serve as a baby-sitter, and I remind the children that they can also have a quiet good time reading or drawing. In this respect, I'm lucky. Because of their numbers, my children usually prefer to play in a social way with each other, rather than simply sitting and watching television. (They'll also have friends get off the school bus with them, so I often have 8, 9, or 10 kids instead of just 5.)

Running lends itself to a kind of "touring" that works very well on family vacations. Running through a city is often the quickest way to get to know it. When Donna Welsh's husband ran in the Boston Marathon, the whole family went along. It was raining when they arrived, but they put on their running gear and ran sightseeing through the Freedom Trail and the rest of Boston. In the country, running on wooded paths and down country lanes can be a beautiful experience for a family group and an opportunity for communication and sharing.

Family participation in races can offer both fun and good feelings of achievement. In many ways my "best" race was the Greenwich 5-Mile Memorial Day Race that I ran with my children last year. I began it not knowing how many of them would finish. There are certainly few adults who could enter a race of that length with as little preparation as the children had, but somehow kids get away with it. Their move favorable ratio of heart and lung size to body weight gives them an aerobic advantage during their growing years. Even so, their training was haphazard at best. Jim and I would take them out on occasional weekends for a two-mile loop, stopping every few hundred yards to allow the stragglers to catch up, and the farthest any of them had run was 3½ miles at a fun event several weeks earlier.

Three of the girls dropped out fairly early, but Zachary and Samantha finished in good form, with me running back and forth between them (to shouts of "Wrong way!" each time). I ran the last stretch with Samantha, taking a bit of time to check her condition. Entering the high school track for the last half-loop, Samantha broke into a semi-sprint and we crossed the finish line holding hands. Minutes later, Zachary finished in fine shape. My most vivid recollection of the day was the moment when I caught sight of Samantha making her way up the last big hill and realized that she was going to go the whole distance. Running the race had been her choice, so finishing it had been her accomplishment, and watching her gave me an incredible sense of elation.

I should say here that I think it's fine for even relatively young children to participate in short races or fun runs on a low-key basis. I don't think children under ten should do anything that requires maximum physical effort, such as a marathon. The precautions about racing in the heat apply more strongly to children — they are more vulnerable to heat exhaustion because their body mass is smaller and they dehydrate more rapidly. Running also should be totally up to the child in terms of what he or she feels motivated to do. Support from the parents should not veer over into pressure.

## Husbands, Wives, and "Crewing"

There's been a lot of discussion about running being a divisive factor in the home. Pictures are painted of the running spouse sprinting away from family responsibilities, leaving emotional chaos behind. In my experience, and the experience of my friends, it's not so much that the running affects the marriage relationship, but that the quality of the relationship lets you work out the running.

Unless there's unhealthy competition between them, the easiest situation is when the husband and wife both run. They may not be able to run together on a daily basis, since both will probably be sharing child and home care at the busy points of the day. Weekends will provide chances for them to run together, however, and the couples I know treasure this time. Little has to be said during the run. The luxury of the private hour together suffices, and in the runs I've had with Jim the sense of companionship was more eloquent than any verbal exchange.

Situations where only one partner runs can also work out well, since most marriages flourish when both husband and wife are free to develop their own potential. The non-running spouse is sometimes bemused by the jargon and bored with the pre-race shenanigans, but tolerant and really pleased about the husband/wife's increased level of fitness.

*Any* combination of circumstances can work for a couple, as long as both parties accept the running as a facet of their lives. Jim's game is tennis, and he puts most of his energy into that, but he's also an athlete on many other levels. Running was part of his life before it became part of mine, and he understands why it's important to me. From the very beginning my sense of delight in the sport was something I could share with him.

Of course it's one thing to give encouragement to a three-mile daily run and another to actively support the completion of a marathon. Jim's been on hand for each of my marathon efforts, helping in so many ways (many of them highly strenuous) that I sometimes think his work was harder than mine. This is known as "crewing" — a crisp term for the crazed level of drink dispensing, broken-field running, and cheering-on that's so supportive during a race.

The 1977 Boston Marathon was a case in point. I hadn't planned to run this event, but I had unexpectedly qualified for it in a previous Long Island marathon and thought I'd give it a try. When Jim and I arrived in Boston two days before the race to share a four-room apartment with friends, we found that eight other people had the same idea. Six people slept in the apartment and four (including Jim and me) slept in a family Winnebago parked outside on a steep Brookline street. The next day we drove the course from Hopkinton back to Boston, and the Sunday traffic made this tedious, as well as psychologically exhausting.

Patriot's Day dawned unseasonably warm for mid-April (we were hoping for temperatures in the 50s, but it hit 80 degrees that day). At 8:45 we drove out to Hopkinton, and while I picked up my number and registration packet, Jim and his friend Mike drove separate cars to the 4-mile point in Ashland. Jim parked the car near a race point and returned in Mike's car to Hopkinton, arriving just in time to accompany me on the half-mile jog to the starting point near the town green. With the crowd massing (no starting line visible, just throngs), we started off at 12 noon and Jim ran close behind to keep me from getting trampled. Going through Ashland, I looked back to see him cut off to the car.

At 1:40 I passed Wellesley at the halfway mark and began to look for Jim, who was to meet me at 15 miles. Jim and Mike meanwhile had driven on Route 9 to just beyond Wellesley, parked the car on the shoulder of the road, and had run a mile to an exit so they could meet the course of the race. At 15 miles, Jim spotted me and darted into the road, running alongside and offering me water from squeeze bottles. I remember wishing fervently that he would stay with me all the way into Boston, but the car was back on Route 9. Jim ran with me for a mile and a half, then doubled back to the car (racing himself, so he would reach the finish line before I did).

While I wound my way through the last 10 miles, Jim followed Route 9 toward Boston, parked 5 miles from the downtown section, and took the trolley into the city to a point about 2 miles from the Prudential Center. He sprinted that last distance and reached the roped-off ramp to the finish line before me.

I arrived at the "Big Pru" totally drained. All my runs had been in the cold, I'd had no experience running long distances in the heat, and I staggered as I approached the finishing ramp with legs that felt like rubber. It's a weird sensation when your brain is sending out signals to your legs and they won't obey. I remember feeling really light-headed and then falling down on the ramp. The crowd was shouting and screaming at me. Jim ran over to help, but was stopped by a big policeman who said, "Laddie, if you touch that woman you're under arrest!" Jim pleaded, "But she's my *wife*." "I don't care who she is," the Law replied, "if you touch her she's disqualified and you go to jail."

I managed to get up and totter forward again, with Jim urging, "Walk. Don't run, Just *walk*." I was so disoriented that I didn't realize I was on the ramp, but I managed to stumble across the finish line in a daze. Jim whisked me off to the first-aid station in the basement of the Prudential Center (which looked like a Crimean War outpost that afternoon). Jim clocked my time at 3:26, but afterward neither one of us could remember whether I'd actually gone through the finishing chute. That confirmation came with my certificate months later.

Jim's help that day was champion "crewing." This degree

of support is clearly beyond the call of husbandly duty, but I'm grateful for it. Jim's presence has added an extra dimension to all my races. Running or not, we feel like a team.

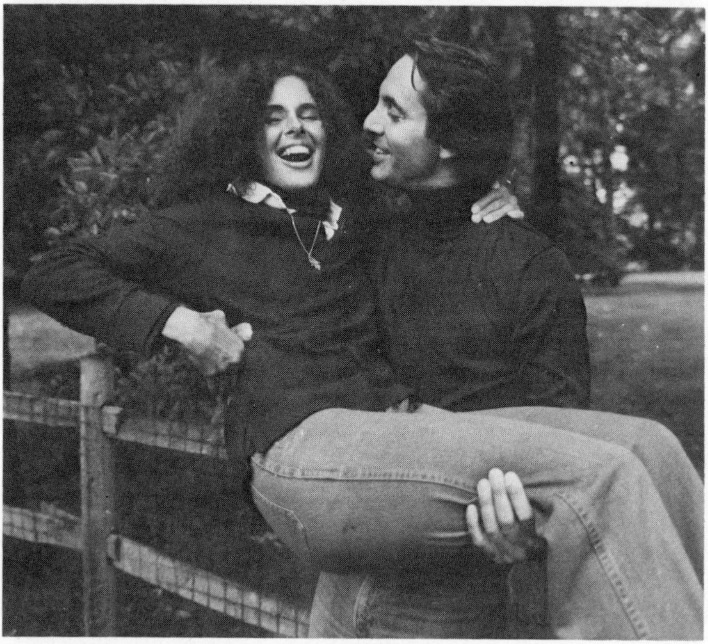

Loving support from Jim. *Ken Regan, Camera 5*

# A Last Word

There are moments when the legendary loneliness of the long distance runner is more than matched by the loneliness of the new mother — or *any* mother at home with young children. Child rearing has its wonderfully funny moments and episodes of tender sharing, but the sense of loneliness can be overwhelming when the volume of work that needs to be done creates an awesome sense of responsibility.

When I began running, I ran for solitude — to have a few moments alone. To my surprise I found a companion out on the road, a friend I'd lost track of during those busy years with the babies. The companion was *me.* I finally had time to slow down and listen to my own breathing, to hear my heart beat and my mind speak.

When I'm running I don't have to make the adjustments and compromises that must — of necessity — rule the rest of my life. Apart from the terrain and weather, the only limitations are those imposed by physical strength. I am free to explore my own avenues, define my own boundaries. Running did not simply help me rediscover that friend — my old self; it took me to new places and showed me new ways to express my thoughts and feelings.

Running creates an inviolate space — one that the runner alone inhabits. The experience is intensely personal; we must explore it for ourselves. I believe running has much to offer anyone who gives her best to the effort. Certainly, for the woman who went from her father's house to school to her husband's door — without ever having a chance to develop her own independence — running can bring particular strengths. Its disciplines and challenges may help a woman truly find herself — and show her that she has untapped reservoirs of power.

# Appendix

# Bibliography

# Appendix

## **Pulse Rate Table** (see p. 49)

The maximum pulse rate (which is the same as the maximum heart rate) is based on the formula of 220 minus the age of the subject. However, the following modifications should be noted:

1. The formula applies more accurately to younger people. With increasing age, the maximum pulse rate tends to drop more slowly than the formula-based one-beat-per-minute rate with each advancing year.

2. Keep in mind that these figures for maximum pulse rate are only approximate; actual heart rates can vary 10–15 per cent in either direction. For individual accuracy it is better to follow the formula that allows you to determine the training rate that is best for you. That is, if you know your own maximum rate (from a stress EKG) and your resting rate (easily measured), then fit these values into the formula:

TARGET RATE = Resting Rate + 75 per cent of the difference between the Maximum Rate and the Resting Rate.

FIGURE I

PULSE RATE TABLE

*Age, Maximal Pulse Rate (MPR), and 70–80 Per Cent Training Effect Range**

| | | Per Cent | | | | Per Cent | | | | Per Cent | |
|---|---|---|---|---|---|---|---|---|---|---|---|
| *Age* | *MPR* | *70* | *80* | *Age* | *MPR* | *70* | *80* | *Age* | *MPR* | *70* | *80* |
| 20 | 200 | 140 | 160 | 39 | 183 | 128 | 146 | 58 | 169 | 118 | 135 |
| 21 | 199 | 139 | 159 | 40 | 182 | 127 | 145 | 59 | 168 | 117 | 134 |
| 22 | 198 | 138 | 158 | 41 | 181 | 126 | 144 | 60 | 168 | 117 | 134 |
| 23 | 197 | 137 | 157 | 42 | 181 | 126 | 144 | 61 | 167 | 116 | 133 |
| 24 | 196 | 137 | 156 | 43 | 180 | 126 | 144 | 62 | 167 | 116 | 133 |
| 25 | 195 | 136 | 156 | 44 | 180 | 126 | 144 | 63 | 166 | 116 | 132 |
| 26 | 194 | 135 | 155 | 45 | 179 | 125 | 143 | 64 | 165 | 115 | 132 |
| 27 | 193 | 135 | 154 | 46 | 177 | 123 | 141 | 65 | 164 | 114 | 131 |
| 28 | 192 | 134 | 153 | 47 | 177 | 123 | 141 | 66 | 163 | 114 | 130 |
| 29 | 191 | 133 | 152 | 48 | 177 | 123 | 141 | 67 | 162 | 113 | 129 |
| 30 | 190 | 133 | 152 | 49 | 176 | 123 | 141 | 68 | 161 | 112 | 128 |
| 31 | 190 | 133 | 152 | 50 | 175 | 122 | 140 | 69 | 161 | 112 | 128 |
| 32 | 189 | 132 | 151 | 51 | 174 | 121 | 139 | 70 | 160 | 112 | 128 |
| 33 | 188 | 131 | 150 | 52 | 173 | 121 | 138 | 71 | 160 | 112 | 128 |
| 34 | 187 | 130 | 149 | 53 | 172 | 120 | 137 | 72 | 160 | 112 | 128 |
| 35 | 186 | 130 | 148 | 54 | 171 | 119 | 136 | 73 | 160 | 112 | 128 |
| 36 | 186 | 130 | 148 | 55 | 171 | 119 | 136 | 74 | 160 | 112 | 128 |
| 37 | 185 | 129 | 148 | 56 | 170 | 119 | 136 | 75 | 160 | 112 | 128 |
| 38 | 184 | 128 | 147 | 57 | 170 | 119 | 136 | | | | |

* *Fractions omitted.*
(From *The U.S. Air Force Academy Fitness Program for Women* by Jack Galub [Englewood Cliffs, N.J.: Prentice-Hall, 1979]).

## **Running Clubs** (see page 66)

NATIONAL JOGGING ASSOCIATION,
919 18th Street, N.W., Washington, D.C. 20006.
(202) 785–8050
President — Lt. Gen. R. L. Bohannon.
Specify: Membership Information, Suite 830.

For the $15 annual membership fee, the NJA will send you

their monthly newspaper, *The Jogger,* which lists races nationwide by state and offers a battery of running information. There is also a 10 per cent discount on running books. The NJA also sponsors various challenge programs and fun runs nationwide. The NJA is a nonprofit group, so membership fees are tax-deductible.

ROAD RUNNERS CLUB OF AMERICA,
1226 Orchard Village, Manchester, Missouri 63011.
President — Jerry Kokesh.
Membership Information: Sanford Schmidt, 3203 Agnes Blvd., Alton, Illinois 62002.
(Send stamped, self-addressed envelope for membership information.)

The RRC is the country's foremost running organization and has over 250 local chapters. The annual fees vary locally from $3 to $15 per year. The at-large membership fee in the national organization (in lieu of a local chapter) is $4. The national membership includes a quarterly newspaper, *Footnotes,* plus some local-chapter privileges (including reduced entry fees for RRC-sponsored races).

## **Basal Body Temperature Chart** (see page 114)

Most women have occasional concerns about their menstrual cycles — worries about lateness, other irregularities, or effective ovulation are common to us all. There is one simple step which may clarify menstrual uncertainties and it requires the simplest equipment: an oral thermometer, a sheet of graph paper, and some patience. The procedure involves keeping an accurate daily record of the basal body temperature (BBT), which is the temperature taken first thing in the morning upon awakening. This is done each day of the menstrual cycle and is familiar to most women who have ever had difficulty becoming pregnant. The BBT chart (see Figure 2) enables them to determine

FIGURE 2

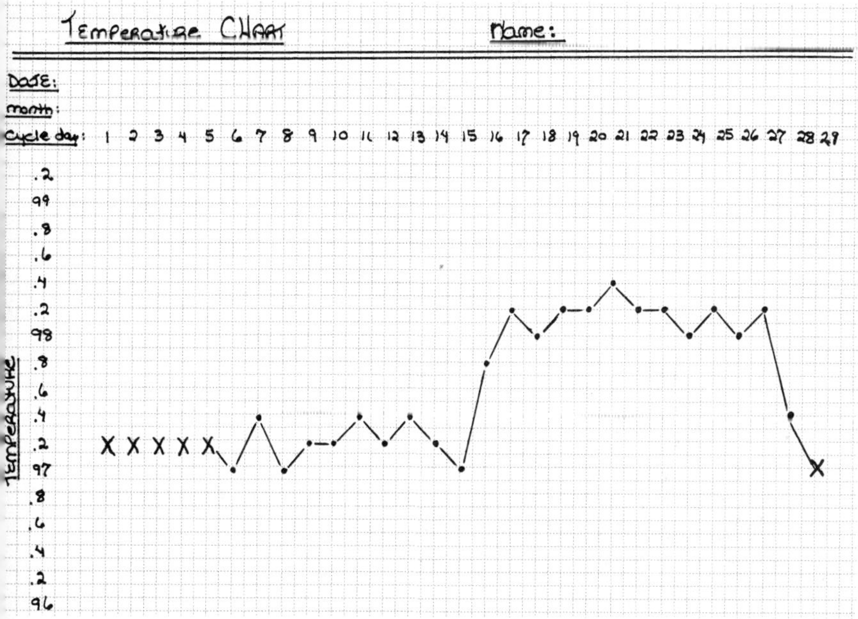


whether failure to ovulate is causing the infertility problem.

Record keeping should begin the first day of the period (day one of the cycle), and x's on the graph paper signify that the period is in progress. Care should be taken to insure the accuracy of the temperature readings — so there should be no eating, drinking, or jumping out of bed before inserting the thermometer, which should stay in the mouth for a full 5 minutes. (If you have difficulty reading an ordinary thermometer, you may want to invest in an Ovulindex, which is a thermometer that magnifies the printed scale: the read-out is in .1 degrees instead of .2.)

The value of the temperature chart is based on the fact that during the second half of the menstrual cycle (that segment between ovulation and the onset of the next period, which is termed "luteal phase"), there is typically a rise of half a degree or more in the BBT. This rise is due to the higher level of progesterone that characterizes the luteal phase, and the temperature remains elevated until a day or so before the next period. According to Dr. Shangold, 90 per cent of ovulatory women will have this rise, and if your temperature chart reflects this biphasic pattern, you may assume your cycle is ovulatory.

When it comes to determining the exact time of ovulation, the temperature chart is not so reliable. Dr. Shangold observes it is generally two or three days after ovulation before the higher progesterone levels are reflected in the temperature rise. If you are trying to pinpoint the time when you are most fertile, the temperature chart will only indicate this in retrospect.

Luteal-phase insufficiency is a subtle hormonal irregularity that may occur in a woman who appears to be menstruating and ovulating regularly. This irregularity can generally be spotted with the help of the temperature chart and occurs when the corpus luteum (literally "yellow body" — the name given to the empty follicle because it turns a bright yellow-orange after the release of the egg at ovulation) fails to produce as much progesterone as it is supposed to. As a result, the uterine lining is not properly primed to support a pregnancy, so that although fertilization may occur, pregnancy does not ensue. Luteal-phase insufficiency also means a shorter luteal phase — the lower progesterone output causes the period to intervene before the usual 14 days.

Dr. Shangold investigated luteal-phase insufficiency in one woman runner whom she monitored continuously throughout 18 cycles and found an inverse relationship between the length of the luteal phase in days and the average number of miles logged on a weekly basis during each cycle. In cycles with a shorter luteal phase, Dr. Shangold also measured lower levels of progesterone. So if the elevated phase of her temperature chart lasts ten days or less, it should alert the runner to the possibility of luteal-phase insufficiency.

Even if you think your temperature chart is inconclusive (the graph line may seem to move up and down at random), don't dismiss the procedure as a futile exercise. An accurate record of your basal body temperature can provide a wealth of information to your physician.

## **Fat Utilization** (see page 148)

J. O. Holloszy et al., "Physiological Consequences of the Biochemical Adaptations to Endurance Exercise," *The Marathon: Physiological, Medical, Epidemiological, and Psychological Studies,* Annals of the New York Academy of Sciences, Vol. 301, 1977, ed. Paul Milvy, pp. 440–50. This article makes the point that the increased utilization of fat as fuel for exercise is entirely due to the adaptive increase (training effect) in muscle mitochondria and the increase in mitochondrial enzymes involved in fatty-acid oxidation, and is not the result of higher concentrations of free fatty acids in the blood, as was originally believed.

Also of interest: Birgitta Essén, "Intramuscular Substrate Utilization During Prolonged Exercise," *The Marathon,* ed. Paul Milvy, pp. 30–44. This article examines the ways different types of fibers found in skeletal muscle rely variously on intramuscular glycogen (i.e., carbohydrate) and triglyceride stores (i.e., fat) as fuel for exercise. Of special interest to the dieter, the author notes that higher work intensities rely more on glycogen for energy, whereas exercise of moderate intensity (i.e., steady aerobic) utilizes more triglycerides — that is, it helps to burn off more fat.

## **Hormonal Changes in Exercise** (see page 153)

H. Galbo, et al., "Hormonal Regulation During Prolonged Exercise," *The Marathon,* ed. Paul Milvy, pp. 72–80. An interesting discussion of the hormonal changes induced by prolonged exercise. It points out the similarity between the pattern of changes induced by prolonged exercise and the pattern of hormonal response to other conditions of glucose deprivation such as fasting and hypoglycemia — that is, decreased concentration of insulin and increased concentration of glucagon, catecholamines, growth hormone, thyroid-stimulating hormone, and corticosteroids. The study suggests that this pattern promotes the mobilization of free fatty acids and stimulates the liver to release stored glucose into the bloodstream for fuel.

# Bibliography

## Good Reading About Running

Albohm, Marge. "Does Menstruation Affect Performance in Sports?" *The Physician and Sportsmedicine,* March 1976.

Bailey, Covert. *Fit or Fat?* Boston: Houghton Mifflin Company, 1978.

Burfoot, Amby. "The Meatless Runner." *Runner's World,* February 1978.

Burger, Robert E. *Jogger's Catalog: The Source Book for Runners.* New York: M. Evans and Company, 1978.

Cooper, Kenneth H. *The New Aerobics.* New York: Bantam Books, 1970.

———. *The Aerobics Way.* New York: M. Evans, 1977.

Costill, David. "Performance Secrets: Coffee Makes Longer Easier" and "Sweeten Races with Sugar." *Runner's World,* July 1978.

Dick-Read, Grantly. *Childbirth Without Fear: The Original Approach to Natural Childbirth.* New York: Harper & Row, 1972.

Erdelyi, G. J. "Effects of Exercise on the Menstrual Cycle." *The Physician and Sportsmedicine,* March 1976.

Falls, Joe. *The Boston Marathon*. New York: Macmillan, 1977.

Feldenkrais, Moshe. *Awareness Through Movement*. New York: Harper & Row, 1972.

Fixx, James F. *The Complete Book of Running*. New York: Random House, 1977.

Galub, Jack. *The U.S. Air Force Academy Fitness Program for Women*. Englewood Cliffs, New Jersey: Prentice-Hall, 1979.

Gerber, E. W., P. Berlin, J. Fleshin, et al. *The American Woman in Sports*. Reading, Massachusetts: Addison-Wesley Publishing Company, 1974.

Glasser, William. *Positive Addiction*. New York: Harper & Row, 1976.

Glover, Bob, and Jack Shepherd. *The Runner's Handbook*. New York: Penguin Books, 1978.

Greist, John H., et al. "Antidepressant Running." *Psychiatric Annals,* Vol. 9, No. 3, March 1979.

Harris, Dorothy V., and Susan E. Jennings. "Self-Perceptions of Female Distance Runners." *The Marathon: Physiological, Medical, Epidemiological, and Psychological Studies*. Annals of the New York Academy of Sciences, Vol. 301, 1977, ed. Paul Milvy, pp. 808–19.

Harrison, Mary. *Infertility: A Guide for Couples*. Boston: Houghton Mifflin Company, 1977.

Herman, Hank. ". . . But Will They Still Be Running in 1989?" *Family Health,* April 1979.

Hittleman, Richard. *The 8 Steps to Health and Peace*. New York: Bantam Books, 1975.

Hlavac, Harry F. *The Foot Book*. Mountain View, California: World Publications, 1977.

Jackson, Ian. *Yoga and the Athlete*. Mountain View, California: World Publications, 1975.

Kostrubala, Thaddeus. *The Joy of Running*. Philadelphia and New York: J. B. Lippincott, 1976.

Lance, Kathryn. *Running for Health and Beauty: A Complete Guide for Women*. Indianapolis and New York: The Bobbs-Merrill Company, 1977.

Lauersen, Niels. *It's Your Body*. New York: Grosset and Dunlap, 1977.

Mandell, Arnold. "The Second Second Wind." *Psychiatric Annals,* Vol. 9, No. 3, March 1979.

Mayer, Jean. *A Diet for Living*. New York: David McKay Company, 1975.

———. "Ten Nutritional Myths." *Family Health,* May 1979.

Milvy, Paul, ed. *The Marathon: Physiological, Medical, Epidemiological, and Psychological Studies.* Annals of the New York Academy of Sciences, Vol. 301, 1977. This is the most thorough study of running to date and is recommended for the reader who wants a full grasp of the more technical aspects of the sport.

Morgan, William P. "Anxiety Reduction Following Exercise." *Psychiatric Annals,* Vol. 9, No. 3, March 1979.

———. "Negative Addiction in Runners." *The Physician and Sportsmedicine,* Vol. 7, No. 2, February 1979.

———. "The Pain Merchants." *Runner's World,* June 1978.

——— with Michael L. Pollock. "Psychologic Characterization of the Elite Distance Runner." *The Marathon: Physiological, Medical, Epidemiological, and Psychological Studies.* Annals of the New York Academy of Sciences, Vol. 301, 1977, ed. Paul Milvy, pp. 382–403.

Sacks, Michael H. "Psychiatric Aspects of Sports." *Psychiatric Annals,* Vol. 9, No. 3, March 1979.

Selye, Hans. *The Stress of Life*. New York: McGraw-Hill, 1956.

Sheehan, George. *Dr. Sheehan's Medical Advice for Runners.* Mountain View, California: World Publications, 1978.

———. *Dr. Sheehan on Running*. Mountain View, California: World Publications, 1975.

———. "Stress Fractures" ("Medical Advice"). *Runner's World*. April 1979.

Spino, Mike. *Beyond Jogging — The Inner Space of Running.* New York: Berkley Publishing Corp., 1976.

Subotnick, Steven I. *The Running Foot Doctor*. Mountain View, California: World Publications, 1977.

Ullyot, Joan. *Women's Running*. Mountain View, California: World Publications, 1976.

## Cookbooks

Braué, John R. *Uncle John's Original Bread Book*. New York: Pyramid Books, 1961.

Ewald, Ellen Buchman. *Recipes for a Small Planet*. New York: Ballantine Books, 1973.

Hewitt, Jean. *The New York Times Natural Foods Cookbook*. New York: Avon Books, 1971.

Hunter, Beatrice Trum. *The Natural Foods Cookbook*. New York: Pyramid Books, 1961.

Lappé, Frances Moore. *Diet for a Small Planet*. New York: Ballantine Books, 1971.

Thomas, Anna. *The Vegetarian Epicure*. New York: Vintage Books, 1972.